BECOMING LEAN *and* FREE

Surprising Secrets to Healthy Weight

KRIS DORAN WILLIAMS, MCHC

Copyright © 2019 by Kris Doran Williams

All rights reserved. No part of this book may be reproduced in any form or by any electronic or mechanical means (including information storage and retrieval systems) without permission in writing from the publisher, except by reviewers who may quote brief passages in a review.

ISBN: 978-0-9995332-1-5 (Paperback Edition)

This book is written using information researched in print and on the internet, as well as information from the author's personal experience. Please check references at the end of the book to verify scientific suppositions and studies.

Scripture is taken from the Holy Bible, NEW INTERNATIONAL VERSION®, NIV® Copyright © 1973, 1978, 1984, 2011 by Biblica, Inc.® Used by permission. All rights reserved worldwide.

Book Design by Kris @ krisgraphics.com
Cover Design by Kris @ krisgraphics.com
Cover Font: Alegreya Sans and Qwigley
Interior Chapter Head Font: Flavors
Interior Body Font: Alegreya

Printed and bound in the USA
First Printing: July 2019

To contact the publisher visit:
www.kriswilliamswellness.com

IMPORTANT CONSIDERATIONS

The ideas, concepts, and opinions expressed in this book are intended to be used for educational purposes only. This book is sold with the understanding that the author and publisher are not rendering medical advice of any kind.

This book is not intended to replace medical advice, nor to diagnose, prescribe, or treat any disease, condition, illness, or injury.

Please be advised that before beginning any diet, exercise, or lifestyle program, including any aspect of the approaches mentioned in *Becoming Lean and Free*, it is important that the reader receive full medical clearance from a licensed physician. The author and publisher claim no responsibility to any person or entity for liability, loss, or damage caused or alleged to be caused directly or indirectly as a result of the use, application, or interpretation of the material in this book.

ACKNOWLEDGEMENTS

I am so grateful to Pat Whitney for her ready and generous spirit in editing this manuscript, to Matt Waymeyer for his biblical overview, and to all of those who read and offered feedback on *Becoming Lean and Free* with enthusiasm.

I also offer grateful thanks to my husband, William, and to my daughter, Rachel, both of whom sacrificed many hours to read and edit first drafts, and for their total support throughout the entire process of "mapping out" this guide.

BECOMING LEAN *and* FREE

Surprising Secrets to Healthy Weight

CONTENTS

Introduction: A Travel Guide	xi
Helpful Words and Phrases	xvii
Day 1: Open the Door To Water	1
Day 2: Close the Door To Sugar	9
Day 3: Should You Call in the Replacements?	33
Day 4: Spicing Up Water	47
Day 5: Surprised By What You're Full Of?	57
Day 6: What's Magnesium Got To Do With It?	67
Day 7: The Secret Garden	77
Day 8: Secret Weapon In The Battle Of The Bulge	93
Day 9: Small Change, Mighty Difference	111
Day 10: One Tiny Medicine Cabinet	121
Day 11: Your Nutrient For Success	131
Day 12: Giving Up…and Starting Over	143
Day 13: Garden Delights	153
Day 14: Party Fiber	163
Day 15: Fat: Eat It To Lose It!	173
Day 16: Fats To Add	189
Day 17: Fats To Subtract	207
Day 18: Fishing For The Right Foods	225
Day 19: Eggs And Dairy	239
Day 20: Time For A Trip To The Range	251
Day 21: Grains, Gluten, & Carbs That Count	269
Day 22: Bonus	281
Resources:	291

x

BECOMING LEAN AND FREE IS... A JOURNEY.

You won't get there all at once.

But if you stay on the path, I promise you *can* get there.

BECOMING LEAN AND FREE IS ALSO... A TRAVEL GUIDE.

Whenever you're on a journey, it's handy to have one.

Whenever you're on a journey to lose weight and experience freedom, it's essential to have a *trustworthy one*.

How can you get to the place you want to go if you don't have all the right information --- set out on a clear pathway?

A *trustworthy health and weight-loss guide* provides information (backed by research) for you to think about, chew on, and digest. It presents simple recipes for foods and drinks to include in your diet. It suggests effective actions to take daily so your mind and body can work together. And it offers ways to call on the power of God, the One who made you, to help you live at peace with your body.

A practical guide like this sure would have come in handy for me years ago. Instead, I followed whatever crazy or trendy advice was out there for losing weight --- rarely thinking about what each option would do to my health.

I counted calories.

I limited calories.

I tried to eliminate as many fats from my diet as I could.

I replaced the fats with a lot of grains, cereals, and bread.

I counted on diet drinks to fill me up and satisfy me.

I counted on diet foods to slim me down and satisfy me.

I used coffee drinks as meal replacements.

I used energy drinks as meal replacements.

I exercised hard --- for a while --- without eating or drinking the right things before or after.

Yet all of these things failed, because deep inside I was out of control.

You see, I was a binge-eater. Sometimes chips would start the party, and a bag would be gone in no time. Having any kind of sugar always set me off. I'd taste a small piece of something sweet --- cake, cookies, ice cream --- and then not be able to stop "tasting." No matter what I told myself or how I planned ahead of time, once begun, an uncontrollable urge overtook me, and I'd finished the whole cake, the full box of cookies, the entire carton of ice cream. I felt hopeless to stop.

If I was out to dinner with friends and refused a dessert while with them ("...because I'm sticking to my diet," I explained), I would come home and eat two...or three...or four...desserts I had hidden there.

After binging of course I'd be sick, just like anybody, and over and over again I would castigate myself. In between the binging, and to feel like I had some semblance of self-control, I'd try not eating anything at all for as long as I could... Then, because everybody has to eat, the cycle would start all over again. You can imagine what that yo-yo-ing did to my health. I lost energy, good skin, and a good attitude. And I still gained pounds.

But something changed along the way.

Something inside of me changed because I asked for help from the One who knew me best...and I began to study nutrition. Those two actions took away my dread for achieving a healthy weight.

Let's face it: just the thought of embarking on a new way of eating can cause your defenses to go up and your stomach to rumble. You dread what's coming.

In fact, I'll bet as you're reading this sentence right now, you're automatically and immediately hungrier than you were a minute ago. You're already missing your favorite foods.

The thing is, I know you're reading this book because you *want* to embark on a new path to a weight that's right for you...but at the same time you *don't want* to...because you *believe* it will be hard to stick to the path.

And you also believe it will require denial...of all the foods you enjoy.

You think you've been down this road before, and you don't hope for too much success. You've already had your hopes for success squashed way too often. Oh, you might have lost a few pounds here and there, but you found them again after you took the road back to eating "in the real world."

Am I right?

Are you beginning to question whether I, as your health and weight-loss travel guide, know what I'm talking about? Maybe you're asking yourself how *anyone* knows what's safe to eat anymore.

Maybe you're wondering if anyone really knows how to get you to the land of healthy weight --- to the territory where you live at peace with your body?

So I'm going to let you know that someone does.

What I have to share with you in this guide is based on research --- research that you can verify yourself by looking at the sources at the back of the book.

What I have to tell you are things that your doctor, the American Medical Association, the National Institutes of Health, your government, food companies, dieticians, and nutritionists should be telling you. But because of medical treatment bias, money, or politics, many refuse to objectively investigate current science and test the evidence.

For instance:

Has your doctor ever told you that eating a low-fat diet could harm you? Probably not. But he or she should have!

Has your doctor ever told you that lowering or eliminating the amount of fat you eat each day could actually cause you to *gain* weight? Probably not. But he or she should have!

Has your doctor given you the latest research on sugars, and how they bring more harm to your body than just causing you to gain weight?

Probably not. But he or she should have!

Has your doctor given you the latest research on diet sodas and the substances they contain, and how they, too, can actually cause you to gain weight?

Probably not. But he or she should have!

With this guide, you'll be able to arm yourself with up-to-date facts regarding:

- What your doctor isn't telling you about the best foods that can help you achieve your weight goal.
- How ingredients that are dangerous --- and counter-productive to losing weight and achieving your desired weight --- hide in the foods you eat.
- When the best times for eating and drinking are.
- Why confusion exists along the paths to the land of health.

With this guide, you'll be able to turn your mind into a tool that works for you rather than against you. You'll be able to turn your body into a machine that works to lose weight, even when you're not actively doing anything.

Here's what you can expect every day you use this guide:

1. You'll receive a choice piece of information that you can count on to be true about your body or the space it occupies. You'll be asked to "munch" on this information all day long. What you munch on will train you to make the right food choices when you eat "in the real world."

2. Each day you'll receive a simple recipe for a food or drink to include in your diet that will help you fight cravings, lose weight, and gain energy.

3. Each day I'm going to request that you do something to get yourself moving. The daily "actions" will at first seem simple, and you may think they're silly. "Ha! What difference is this going to make?" you'll probably ask yourself as you go from day one to day two. But humor me --- just do it! --- and I will humor you. Laughter, after all, is one of the best medicines for health and happiness.

4. Each day I'll suggest a prayer to offer to the God who made you, understands you, has a plan for you, and wants the best for you. He wants to communicate with you to give you hope, help, and the power to successfully reach your destination.

Can you stick with this guide for at least 21 days?

Can you make a 21-day commitment?

The reason why I advise sticking to a plan for at least 21 days is that this is the minimum amount of time most people need to begin to form a habit.

Remember the piece of wisdom that says: Sow an act and you reap a habit. Sow a habit and you reap a character. Sow a character and you reap a destiny.

What do you want for your destiny? Do you want to end up where healthy eating and healthy living happen naturally? Do you want to live in a place where you live at peace with your body? If so, follow this guide for at least 21 days. Find out what it's like to experience power through self-control over your mind and body.

Trust me. You can do amazing things. I know you can, because I am one of you.

BEFORE EMBARKING ON ANY JOURNEY, IT'S HELPFUL TO LEARN A FEW FOREIGN WORDS AND PHRASES.

WORDS TO KNOW BEFORE YOU GO

1. INFLAMMATION

As you go through this guide, you're going to see information related to foods (and components of certain foods) that "fight inflammation" in your body. Perhaps you've always understood inflammation to be a good thing because its a body process that fights bacteria that causes infection. Why should you "fight" or eliminate something that's working to kill harmful bacteria in your system?

Consider this:

You cut your finger while chopping vegetables. Your finger turns red, swells, and gets hot, displaying three common signs of inflammation. These signs indicate that infection-fighting cells have rushed to the site of your injury to prevent bacteria or viruses from taking up residence. Following a normal course of events (i.e., you leave the wound protected and you don't irritate it any further), in a day or two, when the unhealthy bacteria is killed, the swelling will go down, the redness will diminish, and the cut will heal.

In this scenario, inflammation is effective in helping to heal your wound and has done its job well.

When is inflammation a very bad thing?

Inflammation is a very bad thing when it is chronic.

For instance, say you keep cutting the same finger over and over again. Your body, wanting to heal itself, would keep sending messages to your finger that keep it red, swollen, and hot, and the wound would never calm down enough to mend.

This is what happens when you continually irritate your intestinal tract with certain foods or drinks that are known to bring harm to or "inflame" the cell tissues there.

Say you are sensitive to gluten but keep eating gluten anyway. Pretty soon your intestinal tract becomes inflamed and what you experience because of inflammation can be anything from bloating and nausea to constipation, diarrhea, headaches, depression, or brain fog. Or say you regularly eat or drink other foods that contain components which are known to "irritate" specific organs, joints, or nerve tissue. Because you continue to eat or drink these foods, your organs, joints, or nerve tissue never get a chance to calm down and you end up experiencing any number of maladies and diseases --- each dependent on the part of your body the inflammation affects --- including diabetes, asthma, arthritis, Alzheimer's disease, cancer...and obesity.

Inflammation is always present in the person who holds on to excess pounds that aren't eliminated, in the person who can't maintain his or her weight, and in the person who lacks an adequate amount of energy.

Furthermore, not being able to lose weight, not being able to maintain weight, and continually grasping for more energy causes stress. And stress causes even more inflammation in your body.

It's a terrible cycle that's difficult to extricate yourself from.

You've tried to do it alone. Now it's time to reach for outside help.

You need a friend to support you --- a friend who will explain to you the foods that work *for* you --- a friend who will warn you of the foods that work *against* you.

And you need to know the One who created you so you can ask for the necessary support and outside help you need to be free.

(One of the ways to get to know the One who created you is by asking for help. Really. Draw near to Him in your thoughts and through the words He writes. As it is written: "Draw near to God, and He will draw near to you.")

Okay.

So from now on, you can consider me one friend who is passionate about working with you.

In this guide I'm going to share with you information on foods that can work for you, too, to help you lose weight, maintain your weight, and give you the energy you need to think well and move well through your day.

I'm also going to share with you information on foods that work against you.

Foods that work against you are foods that cause chronic inflammation in the lining of your gut or other body cells as you continue to eat them. I'm yearning to expose these dangerous foods to you so that you can be healed. So that you can be made whole again. So that along with a leaner body you can regain your health, energy, and self-esteem.

You may be surprised to find out what these dangerous foods are, by the way.

I want you to know about them so you can exercise power over them. (Knowing your enemy is the first step to conquering your enemy.)

I'm also going to suggest substances that you can add to your diet so that inflammation never even has a fighting chance in the battle of the bulge.

Knowing which foods cause inflammation and which foods fight it are two of the best strategies to reduce chronic inflammation and stay healthy.

Reducing chronic inflammation allows you to absorb only the calories you need and to achieve and maintain the weight you desire.

Use this guide to help you fill up with natural anti-inflammatory foods one day at a time.

2. JUICING

Juicing is the practice of separating out as much liquid as you can from fruits and vegetables. It is an exceptional --- and easy --- way to include in your day all of the "magic" ingredients you need to fight inflammation…and to lose weight and stop your cravings!

You can use a hand-held device to squeeze juice from a lemon or lime, but many fruits and vegetables require a machine to do the work of extraction.

In 1990 the World Health Organization recommended that you eat at least 400 grams (about 14 ounces, or a little less than 1 pound) of fruits and vegetables every day. Australia recommends that their citizens eat 2 fruit servings and 5 vegetable servings a day.

How can you get a pound of fruits and vegetables (or 2 fruit portions and 5 vegetable portions) regularly in your diet?

By juicing them! Dr. Oz says that juicing enables you to "add variety to your diet while helping you get the necessary nutrients from fruits and vegetables."

Of course, he warns that juicing does not mean that you have to completely stay away from solid foods (and juicing is not a substitute for a medical diagnosis or treatment).

You'll notice that I include several liquid recipes on your daily Tasting Menu in this guide.

You can choose to either juice the ingredients, or blend them.

Sipping on freshly made juices --- and especially sipping on blended smoothies --- can make a world of difference in your ability to lose weight and maintain your health.

3. BLENDING:

Instead of extracting the liquid portion from solid fruits and vegetables, a blender chops and swirls all parts of them into a wet pulp --- a "smoothie." Sometimes you might peel the skin or cut away the outer rind of your fruits or vegetables before plopping them into a blender, and you'll almost always have to add water and/or ice. (Vegetables are not often "liquid-y" when blended, and water must be added to turn your blended vegetables into a drink, rather than a pudding. Plus, a blender's machine tends to warm its ingredients, so you might need to add ice to keep the components cold.)

Blending fruits and vegetables allows you to retain --- and so consume --- important fiber, vitamins, and other plant nutrients that often get discarded when the same foods are juiced. For some, getting used to sipping on blended vegetable smoothies is a big adjustment. If you are one of those persons, you can start out by juicing, and your taste buds will gradually adjust to the blended versions.

Go to *www.kriswilliamswellness.com* for more juicing and blending ideas, as well as suggestions for what type of juicer or blender might be best for you to choose.

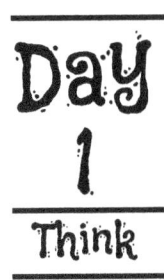

OPEN THE DOOR TO WATER

A journey begins with the first step.

And now that you've taken the first step and found your way to my house, I'm inviting you in.

No doubt you're ready for some refreshment.

What would you like?

Are you hungry? Or thirsty?

Can you tell the difference?

You'll need to know later on when the journeying gets tougher... when you're feeling tired, sluggish, foggy-brained...or think you're hungry.

The truth is, the first thing your body needs when you feel any of those things is...water!

So, would you try an experiment today?

Before reaching for your next meal or snack, would you have a glass of water first?

Your body has big needs --- needs that must be met every day so that it will function smoothly...efficiently...the way it's supposed to function...the way it was created to function.

One of your body's biggest needs is for liquids.

More than one half of your weight comes from them.

Each and every tiny cell that works with every other cell to fill out your whole being requires liquids to function. If you go without liquids for more than three days…you…will…die.

Did you know that the kind of liquids you swallow can affect every tiny little cell in your body positively or negatively? If I were writing a sci-fi drama, I might say that the type of liquid you are transfused with can work for good, or for evil.

But that would be another book.

And since you're sitting in my living room very comfortably without anything to drink, let me pose another question.

If you were thirsty, what would you choose --- right now --- to quench your thirst?

Would you choose a cup of coffee, a can of soda, a glass of fruit juice, an iced tea, a lemonade, an energy drink, a flavored water, a mug of beer, a glass of wine, or a martini (dry, shaken, not stirred)?

Do you recognize that what you choose might not be what makes all those tiny cells very happy? That what you choose to pour into your throat may be the equivalent of pouring unleaded gasoline into a diesel fuel truck, or sludge instead of Draino down your blocked kitchen sink. In the first example, if you drive the truck after putting in the wrong fuel, you'll ruin the engine, and eventually, the engine will just quit; in the second example, the sludge will clog up the sink pipes even more.

What liquid enables your body to function at its optimal level?

You know already that the answer is WATER. Pure, filtered water, or water from a spring.

(Using tests performed on tap water systems throughout the United States between 2010 and 2015, the Environmental Working Group detected an abundance of contaminants that have been linked to cancer, brain and nervous system damage, fertility, fetal or child development problems, and hormonal disruption. To be safe, filtered or spring water is best.)

Water helps to regulate your body temperature, keeps your eyes, nose, and mouth moist, lubricates your spinal cord, and cushions your joints. Enough water in your system helps to prevent kidney stones. Water is necessary to help you digest your meal and remove the waste after digestion is complete. Imagine what your garbage bins look and smell like when you never have the trash removed. Your gut needs water to help you "take out the trash"!

And another thing water is good for?

Losing and maintaining a proper weight.

In fact:

One of the best ways to lose weight (or keep your body at its best weight) is by drinking water --- pure (spring or filtered), life-giving water. Simple, right?

This is your number one secret for losing weight. How can something so simple, inexpensive, and available be so powerful?

Here's how drinking water may help you lose weight:

1. ***Drinking water can help you reduce the total amount of calories consumed daily.***
   The catch is: you've got to replace the lattés, fruit juices, sodas, and other sugar-heavy drinks with...? You got it: pure water.

   And look at the rewards: such a habit could help you reduce your caloric intake by at least 200 calories a day, with very little effort.

2. ***Drinking water can help to reduce your appetite.***
   Research in 2010 showed that adults who drank about 16 ounces (500 milliliters) of water before each meal lost an average of 4.4 pounds (2 kilograms) over three months.

   A more recent study from 2015 confirmed that adults who drank 16 ounces (500 milliliters) of water 30 minutes before each meal lost 3 pounds more weight over 12 weeks than adults who hadn't done so beforehand. By the end of the 12-week study, these adults had lost 9 pounds (4.3 kg), which is about the average amount people lose following popular diets that restrict calories.

3. ***Drinking water throughout the day will increase the amount of energy you use while you rest --- meaning: you burn calories while doing nothing, simply because you drink water!***

Granted, this process may take a while. For instance: in one study women who were overweight and drank more than 34 ounces (1 liter) of water per day lost an extra 4.4 pounds (2kg) of weight during the one-year experiment.

Today's Goal:

Remember your experiment: you are paying attention to your body in order to recognize what thirst feels like. See if you can distinguish the times when you think you are hungry --- from when you are actually thirsty.

Test this. The next time you are "so hungry you could eat a horse," drink a glass of cool, filtered or spring water, then take note of how you feel. Notice that you're not as hungry as you thought you were?

Prepare for Tomorrow's Goal: Please start your day tomorrow by drinking a glass of water --- at a temperature comfortable for you. Drink one glass before each meal and before each snack.

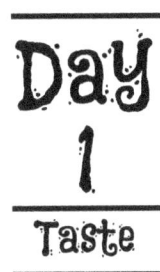

PURE WATER
(Serves 1)

Ingredients:

   12 ounces purified or spring water *(room temperature or slightly chilled)*
   1 fresh lemon or lime wedge

Directions:

- Pour water into a tall glass.
- Squeeze in juice from the lemon or lime.
- Drink 1 glass before each meal or snack.
- Enjoy!

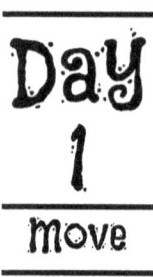

Day 1
move

MOVE YOUR BODY, GROW YOUR RESOLVE
(a movement to help you tune-up --- and get in-tune --- with your body)

BREATHE

Dress in loose, comfortable clothing (or in bedclothes).

Lie on your back on a flat, comfortable surface (or your bed).

Place your hands at your sides.

Close your eyes *and your mouth*.

Breathe in deeply through your nose, then exhale.

Breathe in again. Try to feel your chest rising.

Place your hands on your chest.

Breathe in again, this time slowly, and feel your chest expand. Exhale slowly.

Breathe in again to a count of 4, then exhale to a count of 8.

Now place both hands over your abdominal area.

Inhale again, and allow the air to reach *all the way into your belly*. See if you can feel your abdomen rising.

Breathe in again to a count of 4, then exhale to a count of 8. (Make sure you exhale everything from your belly.)

Do this 10 times.

Today, before you eat, do this belly-breathing exercise 4 times.

Breathing this way helps to wake up your digestion and relax your stomach muscles.

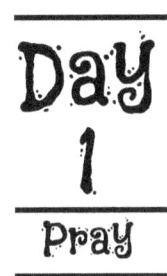

Day 1
Pray

HELLO, GOD...

it's _____ [fill in your first name].

I think you're the Person I should talk to...

because it says in the Bible that you're the One who...

created my inmost being...you knit me together in my mother's womb.

It says there that *you've searched me and you know me.*

You know when I sit down and when I get up;

You know when I go to work and when I'm too sick to get out of bed. In fact, it says you're so familiar with all my ways...

that before a word is on my tongue, you know what I'm going to say.

If you know all this about me, you know when each drop of liquid or morsel of food is on my tongue, too.

You know why I crave things that --- if I eat or drink too much of them --- will make me sick. You know why I refuse to eat or drink so many of the good things you offer.

If it's true that you know me because you made me, help me to know me, too.

 Help me to understand how to eat and drink in a way that honors my body --- and honors you.

Your Word says...

all of your works are wonderful --- and wonderfully made.

If this is true, then you've got to have an explanation for why I've ended up here --- and why I don't feel that this body of mine is so wonderful at the moment.

Psalm 139:1-18

You have searched me, Lord,
and you know me.
You know when I sit and when I rise;
you perceive my thoughts from afar.
You discern my going out and my lying down;
you are familiar with all my ways.
Before a word is on my tongue
you, Lord, know it completely.
You hem me in behind and before,
and you lay your hand upon me.
Such knowledge is too wonderful for me,
too lofty for me to attain.
Where can I go from your Spirit?
Where can I flee from your presence?
If I go up to the heavens, you are there;
if I make my bed in the depths, you are there.
If I rise on the wings of the dawn,
if I settle on the far side of the sea,
even there your hand will guide me,
your right hand will hold me fast.
If I say, "Surely the darkness will hide me
and the light become night around me,"
even the darkness will not be dark to you;
the night will shine like the day,
for darkness is as light to you.
For you created my inmost being;
you knit me together in my mother's womb.
I praise you because I am fearfully and wonderfully made;
your works are wonderful,
I know that full well.
My frame was not hidden from you
when I was made in the secret place,
when I was woven together in the depths of the earth.
Your eyes saw my unformed body;
all the days ordained for me were written in your book
before one of them came to be.

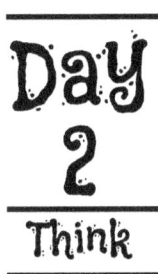

CLOSE THE DOOR TO SUGAR

Good morning! Thanks for stopping by again. Come on inside.

How about a glass of water?

And don't be shy about asking if there's anything to make the water sweeter. I know you're wondering.

You want to know if any of the liquids you've been used to drinking --- a fruit juice, a fruit smoothie, a soda, or an energy drink --- are just as good as water.

You want to know if any of these things are safe to drink if you desire to lose weight, maintain your desired weight, or have more energy.

I understand.

You want to know because water tastes so...bland? You say there's nothing there to make it interesting. You say you can't drink it.

And I say: You're addicted to the sweet taste of alternative drinks.

Can you admit it?

If you can, I'll tell you that your addiction is not really all your fault.

The fault is in ... not your stars ... but the liquids you've been used to drinking. And the foods you've been used to eating.

Water tastes bland because everything you've become accustomed to drinking and eating is spiked up, souped up, and otherwise altered with SUGAR in any or all of its various forms.

Look at the list below.

When you've wanted quick energy in the past, you probably would have reached for something that contained some kind of sugar:

A soda.

A Gatorade.

A fruit juice.

A double caffe latte.

A mocha frappuccino.

A coffee with sugar.

A café con leche.

A bagel.

A muffin.

A candy bar.

An energy bar.

A bowl of cereal.

Sugar is a simple carbohydrate --- and all of the drinks (and foods) above are simple-carbohydrate-rich because they're sugar-rich… and would have provided you with "quick energy."

But I'm guessing you're reading this guide now because something has gone wrong since you started continually reaching for one of the things on the above list.

Your sleep pattern is erratic, and you're tired when the day begins.

You've ended up with headaches, sores, or breakouts on your skin.

You've gotten irritable when you didn't want to, and just when you needed a burst of energy, fatigue set in.

You've ended up with more weight than you need or want, and now aren't able to lose that extra weight, no matter what you try… even if you exercise like crazy.

You've ended up depressed…and feeling somewhat hopeless. You're about ready to give up. You've decided more than once to never go on a "diet" again because you're just going to fail.

And you've gotten angry, too. Why are there so many things to eat or drink at the grocery store that are bad for you? You're wondering why all those fruit juices, fruit smoothies, sodas, energy drinks, bagels, muffins, candy bars, energy bars, or coffees leave you exhausted by dinnertime.

Am I right?

And that's why I've written this guide. Because you're wondering.

So for the next few minutes, stay with me. Don't leave me now, because understanding this next bit of information could give you an understanding of your body and the way it works that could change the rest of your life.

If you know that something is dangerous for you --- for your body, your mind, your emotions, your spirit --- would you still go toward it, want it, touch it, eat it?

Of course you would. That's how you're wired…

as a result of what Eve did in the Garden of Eden. Eve was told that she should not eat fruit from the tree in the middle of the Garden. Eating it (and disobeying the command) would certainly fracture her relationship with God (who made her and gave her the command). Eating it might also ruin her relationship with her husband or possibly make her sick. She went for it anyway. It was so appetizing to look at, and Eve concluded it would be so good to taste. There were other trees in the Garden for her to eat from, even one she was explicitly told would bring her life. But she chose to eat from the tree that was forbidden, the one that would bring her harm.

And that's how it is now for you and me, too. When something is appetizing to look at, we reach for it. When we find that it's sweet to the taste, we go back for it again and again. Even when what we reach for doesn't satisfy our hunger or make us smarter. Even when what we reach for continues to make us sick and tired, causes us to be irritable, and gives us all kinds of diseases. Even when what we reach for provides a direct pathway to making us fatter and fatter. Even though -- -and maybe even because --- we're left emotionally debilitated, we continue to reach for it. Again and again.

If you are a student of the Bible, you may be thinking that as a part of humankind which now lives outside the Garden, the Lord gives you the freedom to eat or drink anything according to your own conscience. "Everything is lawful for me," you'll protest, and I wouldn't argue with you on that. But I would gently remind you of the second part of 1 Corinthians 6:12 which says that "not everything is beneficial." And the Scriptures also warn that you shouldn't allow anything to gain control over your life.

Sugar (and products made from it) may be appealing to your eyes and promise satisfaction, but it (and the products made from it) can definitely gain control over your life.

How?

By making it hard for you to stop consuming it! Sugar lurks everywhere, even in the most unlikely places.

For instance, would you ever think your health could be in jeopardy from consuming not only what you buy from grocery store aisles, Starbucks coffee nooks, or ice cream emporiums, but also in health food shops?

Sugar seems so innocent. It's put in foods and drinks to make you like what you're consuming. To make sure you come back for the same products again and again. Sugar makes you feel good --- at first.

But it triggers damaging processes in your body --- perhaps more than any other food additive. It triggers processes that you usually don't see the results of right away. Be assured though, that the consequences of consuming sugar in excess will eventually lead to the demise of your health and weight.

Deceptive sugar.

Why is this so?

If you're wondering why something that tastes so good could be so harmful, I'll tell you.

It's because of this one truth:

Sugar is not a food.

Sugar is a drug.

"Pure, white, and deadly," John Yudkin called it in his book of the same name. Sugar is just as addictive as heroin or alcohol, but the manifestations of sugar consumption are far more subtle.

Who would have thought that any substance in your food supply would have the ability to mess not only with your body but also with your mind, as well as with your spirit? Who would have thought that any food substance could possess such power?

Deception is powerful, and any substance that can control you without your wanting it to is deceptive.

Do you want to bring saneness, relief, self-control, and real energy back into your life again? If so, you've got to be released from the power of deception. If you desire saneness, relief, self-control, and real energy in your life again, you've got to be freed from the control of sugar.

What's the first step?

Exposing yourself to the truth about sugar --- truth based on science, as well as experience. Knowing the truth is powerful because knowing the truth can set you free. Knowing the truth about sugar starts with some basic facts about food: why you need it, and what the best sources are.

You need food because food provides the fuel your body requires to breathe, to think, to move, to work, and to live.

The three major components of food that provide energy are carbohydrates, proteins, and fats, and all three are necessary for your body's growth and health.

As it turns out, sugar is one of the building blocks of carbohydrates.

That's right...!

Sugar!

Right there inside carbohydrates, one of those three essential sources of energy! Molecules of sugar are used to form both simple and complex carbohydrates.

Now you're probably saying quietly to yourself (and shouting out loud to me): "See! It's right there! Sugar is meant for me to enjoy! Sugar is good! Surely a crucial source of energy that God gave me can't be all bad?"

And I'm going to tell you that you're right.

A carbohydrate is an appropriate source of energy.

But a carbohydrate becomes an inappropriate source of energy when you consume it in its **simple** form --- instead of in its **complex** form.

And now that your voice is calm again, you're going to ask what a simple carbohydrate is, and I'm going to tell you.

A simple carbohydrate is composed of one or two molecules of sugar. A simple carbohydrate is broken down very rapidly in your body --- and an excess amount of it can cause your body a lot of havoc.

Glucose and fructose are simple carbohydrates; each is made up of one molecule.

Sucrose, or white table sugar, is a simple carbohydrate made up of two molecules: one molecule of glucose and one molecule of fructose. (Fructose by itself is roughly one-and-a-half times sweeter than sucrose.)

High fructose corn syrup --- or HFCS --- is a simple carbohydrate, too. High-fructose corn syrup is made from glucose and fructose but contains a higher percentage of fructose than glucose.

A complex carbohydrate is made up of sugar or starch molecules in long complex chains. Complex carbohydrates include whole plant foods (like vegetables), unrefined grains (like brown rice or whole oats), legumes (like lentils or peanuts), roots (like beets and carrots), tubers (like potatoes), and fruits. These carbohydrates are more valuable to your health than simple carbohydrates because the sugars and starches in them may be mixed with protein, fat, vitamins, minerals, and/or a beneficial amount of soluble and non-soluble fiber.

During digestion, complex carbohydrates are broken down *slowly* into the smaller molecules of glucose and fructose that your body uses for energy.

Some complex carbohydrates contain more glucose than fructose, other carbohydrates contain more fructose than glucose.

Here's what happens when you eat complex carbohydrates (containing more glucose than fructose):

- Glucose increases the production of a hormone in your body known as insulin. Insulin does at least three things that are very important to understand if you want to be released from sugar cravings:

  1. Insulin causes your body to suppress the release of *ghrelin*, a hormone that stimulates your appetite and promotes fat storage. If you're trying to lose weight, you don't want anything to stimulate your appetite, nor do you want to put more fat into storage. So eating foods that suppress the release of ghrelin would be a good thing. Eating a glucose-rich food --- fruit, vegetables, yogurt, any kind of bread, rice, or pasta --- will make your body release a lot of insulin into your blood. If your hormones are working correctly, the insulin will cause a decrease in the production of ghrelin and you should feel "full" and satisfied.

  2. Insulin causes your body to increase the release of *leptin*, a hormone whose primary role is to control the energy balance in your body. Leptin, manufactured by your fat cells, is supposed to tell your brain that you don't need to eat more food because you have enough fat stored for energy use. If your hormones are working correctly, the more fat you have, the more leptin your fat cells will produce. The more leptin your cells produce, the "louder" the message will be that tells your brain, "We have enough. You don't have to eat any more."

  3. Insulin helps control the amount of sugar in your blood, which keeps your energy from spiking and crashing.

Here's what happens when you eat a fructose-rich carbohydrate:

- Fructose functions quite differently than glucose in your body. Eating fructose does not stimulate insulin or leptin production, and it does not suppress ghrelin. (This means that eating tablespoons of sugar --- each of which is 50% fructose --- might never leave you feeling like you're satisfied or no longer hungry.)

- Fructose is metabolized almost entirely in the liver,* directly into fat. In fact, fructose is metabolized in the liver in almost the same manner as alcohol. People who drink too much beer get a "beer belly," and people who consume too much fructose get a "fructose belly." High amounts of fructose can also lead to fatty liver disease, scarring of the liver, non-alcoholic liver cirrhosis, and ultimately the need for a liver transplant. (Some beginning signs of liver disease include yellowing of the eyes and skin, swelling in the legs and ankles, itchy skin, nausea, vomiting, and chronic fatigue.)

A new study published in Cell Metabolism in February 2018 suggests that minimum amounts of fructose are transformed into glucose in the small intestine, but when the small intestine is overwhelmed with fructose, the extra amounts travel to the liver for metabolism.

- Besides liver disease, consuming an excess amount of fructose promotes high blood pressure, oxidative stress, depletion of vitamins and minerals, metabolic syndrome, arthritis, gout, cancer, inflammation, and...obesity.
- Fructose interferes with the balance of magnesium in your body, causing bone loss and preventing healthy weight maintenance.
- Fructose is NOT the preferred energy source for your muscles OR your brain. Your brain and blood cells prefer glucose. (Although it's also been shown that your brain can use fat, which we'll talk about down the road.)

Now here's what happens when you consume too many simple carbohydrates composed of glucose and fructose that aren't partnered with proteins, fats, or fibers. In other words, here's what happens when you consume too much sugar in general:

Excess sugar causes your brain to go into frenzy mode. Your hormones get overworked. Excess sugar prevents your body from adequately responding to insulin, ghrelin, and leptin, and will ultimately cause you to become insulin-resistant, ghrelin-resistant, and leptin-resistant.

Surprisingly, studies show that it is not glucose which creates an imbalance in hormones. It is fructose that creates the imbalance. (But sadly, glucose rarely appears alone in foods; its most constant companion is fructose.)

Your body does need small amounts of fructose to break down the glucose you've previously eaten and your body has put into storage. The glucose that sits in storage --- in your liver, skeletal muscle, or fat cells --- is called glycogen, and the more glucose-containing foods you eat, the more glycogen you have in storage.

Remember that white table sugar --- formed into crystals that look so pure and innocent --- contains 50% glucose and 50% fructose... and nothing else. No fiber, no vitamins, no minerals come with it.

It has nothing to offer but empty calories.

It affects your brain like a drug; it affects your body like a drug.

It is a drug.

Too many of the foods available in today's food supply have added sugars, often with their fiber, minerals, and vitamins processed right out of them. Plus, what scientists have learned is that it is the added amounts of *fructose* which appear in the majority of processed foods and drinks today that put your body, mind, emotions, and spirit at extreme risk.

Since fructose does not increase the production of insulin (which regulates the amount of sugar in your blood), when you continually consume fructose-sweetened foods or drinks, your energy will continually spike and crash. You may enjoy the quick fix, but afterward you end up experiencing rapid heartbeats, chest pains, and headaches --- then low energy, difficulty sleeping, and general fatigue. Habit makes you go back for more fructose-sweetened (or other sugar-sweetened) drinks and food, which add more calories, more weight, and keep you addicted to this fructose/sugar cycle.

Including a lot of sugar in your diet doesn't just make you feel a little tired or cause you to gain a little weight, however.

Sugar is the great deceiver. It promises to increase your energy, but because of the havoc it plays with your hormones, you end up decreasing the amount of energy your body can produce in the long run. Sugar doesn't give. Sugar takes. Sugar is a thief.

So if you're trying to lose weight, trying to maintain your weight, or merely trying to increase the amount of energy you have so you can do more things, the following are two truths that --- if you take the time to implant them in your brain --- will bring success to all of your weight and energy efforts:

Truth #1:

Excess sugar = loss of energy.

Truth #2:

Excess sugar = more fat production.

And if you think fat is making you fat, look at the second truth again.

Excess sugar = more fat production.

But:

What if you don't drink sodas?

What if you don't drink fruit juices?

What if you take your coffee black...

and you're still gaining weight...?

Then it's crucial to find out where this sugar criminal hides, and how added amounts of it continually sneak their way into your diet to cause you harm. Manufacturers often give it fancy names to dress it up, like a wolf in sheep's clothing.

Here's how to recognize sugar by its nicknames, which are sugars that get a failing grade:

- **White Table Sugar and White Granulated Sugar**: the two names for "sucrose" that you heard about at the beginning of today, consisting of 50% glucose and 50% fructose.

Sucrose is extracted from sugarcane or sugar beets and refined into crystals.

- **White Powdered Sugar**: a more refined white granulated sugar, also known as confectioners' sugar.
- **Invert Sugar**: a liquid mixture of glucose and fructose that is sweeter than sucrose because of its higher fructose content.
- **Evaporated Cane Juice**: made from boiled cane sugar just as white sugar is, but unlike white sugar, it retains traces of molasses.
- **Light Brown Sugar/Turbinado/Demerara Sugar**: a minimally refined, dry, raw cane sugar lightly coated with molasses. Contains up to 4.5% molasses.
- **Dark Brown Sugar**: refined white sugar with molasses added to it; contains more molasses than turbinado sugar --- up to 6.5%.
- **Barbados/Muscovado Sugar**: produced solely from the sugarcane plant with the nutrient-rich molasses left intact. Can contain up to 10% molasses.
- **Sucanat**: an unrefined sugar made from crystallized pure cane sugar. Contains up to 10% molasses.
- **Brown Rice Sugar**: made from enzymes added to cooked whole-grain rice which allow the rice's starch to break down into maltose, maltotriose and a small amount of glucose. Beware of this sweetener! Brown rice naturally contains the poison arsenic, and brown rice syrup has been shown to contain concentrated amounts of it.
- **Agave**: refined from the agave plant. Agave nectar in its unrefined, natural state does contain compounds known as *fructans* that benefit metabolism and proper insulin regulation. But the heat and enzymes used in refining agave nectar transform the fruct**ans** into fruct**ose**. The result of refining is a sugar content that's 70% fructose! This amount of fructose is higher than the amount in

HFCS, and a dangerous choice because of the way fructose makes it harder for your body to use insulin effectively. Another reason (besides the fructans) agave is often mistakenly advertised as healthy is because it has a low Glycemic Index. The Glycemic Index is a measure of how quickly sugar in a food enters your bloodstream. If sugar enters quickly, you get a "spike" in your blood sugar. The more and higher the spikes, the worse it is for your health. Agave doesn't cause a steep spike in your blood sugar because most of it is fructose, which heads right to your liver (although current research says your small intestine may be involved first). The failure to recognizes fructose metabolism is one reason why the Glycemic Index is not a valid measurement for the healthiness of a food.

- **High-Fructose Corn Syrup (HFCS):** manufactured from corn starch and composed of 55% fructose, 42% glucose, and 3% other sugars or glucose chains. HFCS is pervasive in our current food supply. What makes it so dangerous is its high content of fructose. (Beverages sweetened with HFCS have been tested and shown to contain sometimes 50% more fructose than glucose --- much higher than the ratio of 55% fructose to 42% glucose, which is what manufacturers say is the ratio.) HFCS has been added generously to soft drinks, coffees, teas, sports drinks, cereals, meal bars, energy drinks, cookies, cakes, pies, breads...

The beginning of defeating an enemy is having a positive ID.

Sometimes manufacturers will use other deceptive names for their sugar ingredients like: pure cane sugar, corn sweetener, corn syrup, corn syrup solids, crystal dextrose, evaporated cane juice, fructose sweetener, fruit juice concentrates, liquid fructose, raisin syrup, ribose rice syrup, rice malt, rice syrup solids, Florida crystals, maltodextrin, malted barley, and malts. There are almost 100 different names for sugar and sugar alcohols on ingredient lists.

If you see any of these listed, please beware.

Even if a manufacturer uses "pure, organic cane juice," it's still sugar, and sugar is not your friend.

Sugar is your enemy.

Do you want to be free from addiction to it?

Do you want to lose weight and never find it again?

Do you want to regain your sanity?

Do you want your energy back?

Do you want to gain control of your life?

Then limit the amount of added refined carbohydrates and sugars you allow in your diet. (In fact, if you strictly limited all refined grains and added sugars, you would lose all the weight you wanted or needed to lose.)

How much is too much sugar?

In the early 1900s Americans added an average of 4 teaspoons (16 grams) of sugar to their daily diet.

Today an American adult consumes an average of 19 teaspoons (76 grams) of added sugar every day, and an average child consumes over 32 teaspoons (128 grams). One study concluded that half of all Americans take in 53 teaspoons (212 grams) of sugar a day.

Now here's the kicker:

The Food and Drug Administration's (FDA) current recommendation is that Americans limit their added sugar intake to no more than 10 percent of daily calories.

So if you're eating 2,000 calories a day, then you're "allowed" 200 calories of added sugar each day. That's about 12 1/2 teaspoons, or 50 grams, of sugar per day.

Here's the math:

1 gram of sugar = 4 calories

4 grams of sugar = 1 teaspoon of sugar

4 grams of sugar (1 teaspoon) = 16 calories

50 grams of sugar (12 1/2 teaspoons) = 200 calories

My take: The FDA is like a wild and crazy aunt, the kind who pretty much lets you do whatever you want.

The American Heart Association suggests limiting added sugar even more: to no more than six teaspoons (about 25 grams, or 100 calories) per day for women, and no more than nine teaspoons (36 grams, 144 calories) per day for men.

My take: The Heart Association is like a very kind grandmother; it's being way too easy on you.

Nutritionists --- the kind of people who are really looking after your health --- recommend that if you're at risk of heart disease, cancer, Type 2 Diabetes, or if you're overweight: cut down your added sugar intake to 10-15 grams (or about 2-4 teaspoons per day).

My take: why include any added sugars at all, especially during this 21-day journey with me?

Eventually --- after you've gone through this guide and arrived at your desired weight and energy --- you may want to include (with caution) the following types of sugars that get a passing grade and can be used in a healthy diet. The reason you are justified in using the following types of sugars in small portions is that they contain micronutrients --- vitamins, minerals, amino acids, and fatty acids --- that are beneficial:

- **Blackstrap Molasses**: a byproduct of the sugar-making process. Generally, sugarcane is used to make molasses for human consumption, and sugar beets are used to make molasses for animal feed. About 50% of molasses is sugar: 30% sucrose, 20% invert sugar (invert sugar is about 11% fructose and 9% glucose). 20% of molasses is water, and the rest is composed of ash, proteins, amino acids, fiber particles, chlorophyll, and other earthy matter. Molasses is high in minerals and B-vitamins. In particular, it is a useful source of magnesium, iron, calcium, copper, zinc, and potassium.
- **Sweet Sorghum:** another name for molasses in the southern part of the US.
- **Treacle**: another name for molasses in the UK.

- **Corn Syrup**: manufactured from corn starch and nearly 100% glucose; some brands add HFCS, so it's important to read ingredient labels, and not choose those labeled with HFCS.
- **Honey**: essentially a highly concentrated water solution of glucose and fructose. Depending on the type, honey contains approximately 38% fructose, 31% glucose, 7% maltose, 2% sucrose, 17% water, and a mixture of vitamins, minerals, and amino acids in varying amounts. *Because of the nutrients it brings, honey is an allowable sugar, but only in small quantities (1 teaspoon a day). Choose Manuka honey or a honey local to you which is raw and unfiltered.*
- **Coconut Sugar**: also known as coco sugar, coconut palm sugar, coco sap sugar or coconut blossom sugar and is produced from the sap of the flower bud stem of the coconut palm tree. Coconut sugar contains minerals (potassium, magnesium, iron), short-chain fatty acids, polyphenols and antioxidants that may provide some health benefits. Coconut sugar also includes a fiber called *inulin*, which may slow down the absorption of glucose into your cells, and may explain why this sugar is marked with a lower glycemic index than white table sugar.

  Depending on the content of the minerals, fatty acids, polyphenols, antioxidants and inulin, 70%-79% of coconut sugar is sucrose. The varying percentages depend on the quality of the palm flowers and the process of extracting the sugar from the flowers. *(In spite of its beneficial components, coconut sugar is still sugar. Please eat sparingly.)*
- **Maple syrup**: made from the sap of maple trees with a content of approximately 66% sucrose. The remaining 34% is made up of calcium, potassium, iron, zinc, manganese, and small amounts of additional glucose and fructose.

These were ingredients your grandmothers or great grandmothers used in their dessert recipes --- before the United States was overwhelmed with obesity and cancer --- and in foods that were eaten on special occasions.

Today's Goal (Part-A):

Check your cupboards and remove all bottles, cans, and packaged food you have stored there. Read the labels of every food and drink you've bought. Search your refrigerator, too, and check out the labels of salad dressings, soups, yogurts, sports drinks, protein drinks, energy drinks, and "health" bars. Note any of the following from each label:

- Sucrose
- Fructose
- White Table Sugar
- White Granulated Sugar
- White Powdered Sugar
- Invert Sugar
- Evaporated Cane Juice
- Light Brown Sugar
- Turbinado
- Demerara Sugar
- Dark Brown Sugar
- Barbados Sugar
- Muscovado Sugar
- Sucanat
- Brown Rice Sugar
- Agave
- High-Fructose Corn Syrup (HFCS)
- Pure Cane Sugar
- Corn Sweetener
- Corn Syrup *(If the label doesn't explicitly say that it has no fructose, it most likely has fructose added to it.)*
- Corn Syrup Solids
- Crystal Dextrose

- Evaporated Cane Juice
- Fructose Sweetener
- Fruit Juice Concentrates
- Liquid Fructose
- Raisin Syrup
- Ribose Rice Syrup
- Rice Malt
- Rice Syrup Solids
- Florida Crystals
- Maltodextrin
- Malted Barley
- Malts

Today's Goal (Part-B):

Take note of the grams of sugar each serving contains.

For instance: how many grams of sugar are in a can of Coca-Cola? Or in a serving of breakfast cereal?

You'll see that one 12-ounce can of regular Coke contains 9 and 1/3 teaspoons (38 grams) of total sugar (almost as much as your crazy aunt would allow you to have in one day).

An 8.3-ounce Red Bull Energy Drink contains about 7 teaspoons (28 grams) of sugar.

One tablespoon of Smucker's Strawberry Jam contains 3 teaspoons (12 grams) of sugar. (Imagine loading your toast with 3 teaspoons of sugar?)

One-half cup of Francesco Rinaldi Traditional Pasta Sauce, Original contains almost 3 teaspoons (11 grams) of sugar (and most people eat more than ½ cup of spaghetti sauce).

You'll be surprised to find how much sugar has been added to foods you never would have guessed, and how many clever ways extra sugar is disguised and/or promoted in foods you would expect to be naturally sweet enough, without the need for added sugars.

Sugar is added because manufacturers know that sugar is addictive. They use sugar to lure you back into their Hansel-and-Gretel-cottages-of-packaged-and-processed foods again and again.

Today's Goal (Part-C --- if you are brave):

Eliminate as much sugar from your refrigerator and cupboards as you can. (If you eat cereal, choose brands that have no more than 6 grams of added sugar per serving, and at least 3 grams of fiber and 3 grams of protein.)

The reason I suggest eliminating as much sugar as possible from your diet --- and from your kitchen --- is because of what you've been hearing during our time together: sugar is addictive, every bit as addictive as drugs and alcohol can be.

The more you eat or drink of it, the more you crave, just as you crave more of anything you're addicted to. And the more you have available in your refrigerator or cupboards, the easier it is to reach for it.

Do you want to break your addiction? Do you want to be free?

Refusing to consume sugar is one way to help you break your addiction, and it's much easier to refuse sugar if it's not lurking in your refrigerator or cupboards.

Today's Goals (Part-A through Part-D) comprise step two on your journey to freedom. (Drinking water is step one.)

Soon enough you're going to learn more ways to crush your sugar cravings.

And little by little, you're going to experience freedom --- the freedom of self-control. You'll experience the freedom to reject what is harmful to you and choose what is helpful.

For now --- when sugar is like a spoiled dog snapping at your heels, demanding that you eat it --- drink a glass of water, then choose to eat a whole piece of fruit, or, if you're daring, a whole carrot with a bit of almond butter.

I will be praying that you are strong enough to do these two things.

Give yourself time to adjust.

One glass of water in the morning, one before lunch, and one before dinner. (If you're exercising, drink more.)

Wanting a snack in the middle of the morning or afternoon?

Make a pact with yourself to have a glass of water first.

Then see if you feel better for it.

Is water really your best bet for liquid refreshment?

Yes. But there are options you can substitute here and there.

Try sparkling or mineral water.

If you've been led to believe that all carbonated drinks --- including sparkling/mineral water --- leech calcium from your bones and corrode your teeth, let me guide you along a road less traveled.

While it's true that carbonated water has a bit more acidity than plain water, a study published in 2001 shows that carbonated water will not damage tooth enamel in any significant way. It specifies that even though sparkling mineral water has a slightly more erosive effect on teeth than still water, the impact was 100x less than what carbonated soda has on teeth.

So don't be discouraged.

Today's Goal (Part-D):

Spice up your water by adding a squirt of lemon or lime to your glass. And tomorrow we'll talk about another alternative.

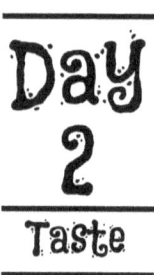

Day 2
Taste

SPARKLING WATER
(Serves 1)

Ingredients:

12 ounces chilled, unsweetened, sparkling water *(for example: Perrier, Pelligrino, Gerolsteiner, Topo Chico, Canada Dry club soda, or Schweppes club soda. No tonic water, please, because of its content of added sugar.)*

1 fresh lemon or lime wedge

Directions:

- Pour sparkling water into a tall glass.
- Squeeze in juice from the lemon or lime.
  (A few times a day, you can replace your purified or spring water with sparkling water.)
- Drink and enjoy!

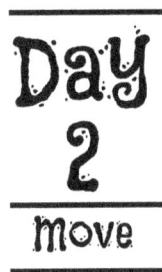

STRETCH

Dress in loose, comfortable clothing (or in bedclothes).

Lie on your back on a flat, comfortable surface (if you lie on your bed, lie at an angle).

Reach your arms over your head.

Grasp one hand with the other.

While holding your hands, squeeze your upper arms against your ears.

Bring your arms back down to your sides and relax.

Next:

Point both of your toes and reach with them as far away from your waist as you can.

Relax.

Next:

Once more: Reach your arms over your head ---

Grasp one hand with the other ---

While holding your hands, squeeze your upper arms against your ears ---

AND

Point both of your toes and reach with them as far away from your waist as you can.

Stretch your arms and your legs away from the core of your

body for as long as you enjoy the release!

Next:

Stretch your arms out to your sides.

Open your legs into a V formation as far apart as you can.

Reach with your arms out to your sides as far as you can,

while:

Pointing your toes and reaching with them as far away from your waist as you can.

Relax.

Do each stretch two or three times.

Today, before you eat, remember to breathe deeply, and then, while standing, stretch your arms over your head and squeeze your arms against your ears.

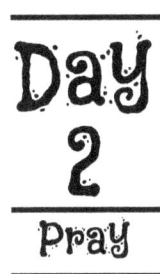

Day 2
Pray

ABOUT THOSE RULES...

Hello, God,

You set up rules for Adam and Eve about what they could and couldn't eat in the Garden of Eden. But here --- outside the Garden --- you said that I'm free to eat according to my own conscience.

Will you help me be conscientious, then, as I explore the information set before me in this guide so that what is helpful for losing unhealthy weight becomes less confusing?

I'm not very good at sticking to an eating plan.

I've been known to mess up.

Foods tempt me, and I give in.

Parties captivate me, and I overindulge.

I promise myself that I'll do one thing, but then end up doing what I don't want to do.

I get out of control.

And I don't know how to stop myself.

Afterward, I feel so embarrassed...so depressed...and so like a failure. And these feelings make me not want to continue with any plan at all!

Up until now, I haven't talked to anyone when I feel out of control like this.

But I'm trusting that I can talk to you.

I'm asking for wisdom.

Help me --- deep in my inmost being --- to understand during these coming days, why certain foods and beverages are good for me, so that I can welcome them into my diet. Help me to understand why certain other foods and drinks are harmful to me, so that I can crowd them out of my diet.

James 1:5-8

*If any of you lacks wisdom, you should ask God,
who gives generously to all without finding fault,
and it will be given to you.
But when you ask, you must believe and not doubt,
because the one who doubts is like a wave of the sea,
blown and tossed by the wind.
That person should not expect to receive anything from the Lord.
Such a person is double-minded
and unstable in all he/she does.*

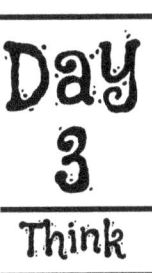

SHOULD YOU CALL IN THE REPLACEMENTS?

You're still wondering, I know, if there's a way to cheat the system. You're wondering if there's a way to satisfy your sweet tooth and continue to remain healthy. Could you, should you, just substitute artificial sweeteners whenever and wherever sugar is lurking? I know I certainly wondered.

If you can't or shouldn't have the real thing, then why not satisfy your sweet tooth with fake sugar? If sugar is harmful, then surely artificial sweeteners are better for you than the real thing...right?

Diet drinks became very popular in the 1970s and 1980s, and even now a majority of people who want to lose weight decide to substitute diet sodas and diet sweeteners for sugared sodas and sugared foods.

How about you? Are you following the crowd by substituting artificial sweeteners for sugar in your beverages and foods, thinking that's a healthier way to go?

I followed the crowd.

I was a diet-soda junkie. With it I thought I was molding my body into better health. I was hoping that with the artificial sweeteners I'd lose weight, get the pick-me-up from the caffeine, and generally keep myself free of disease because I was shielding my organs from sugar.

What I didn't know?

The truth about artificial sweeteners.

That the aspartame in juices, shakes, soft drinks, coffees, teas, and desserts has never been proven to be safe. In fact, it's been proven to be just the opposite.

I was not losing weight and gaining energy by avoiding sugar and using artificial sweeteners --- I was gaining weight, losing energy, and losing my health!

Dr. Mercola writes that all artificial sweeteners are harmful in one way or another. These include:

- Aspartame (NutraSweet, Equal)
- Sucralose (Splenda)
- Saccharin (Sweet 'N Low)
- Acesulfame potassium (Acesulfame-K)

In fact, artificial sweeteners can even be worse than sugar or fructose. In his book, *Sweet Deception (2006)*, Dr. Mercola describes how aspartame continues to appear in diet soft drinks and other diet foods even though it has displayed (so far) the most evidence for harmful effects. Aspartame has been shown to cause cancer (leukemia, lymphoma, and other tumors), yet some soft drink companies continue to promote its "safety."

In his book, *Excitotoxins: The Taste That Kills (1997)*, Dr. Russell Blaylock explains how flavor-enhancers (like MSG, aspartame, and similar substances) added to your foods and drinks can cause harm to your brain, affect your nervous system, and lead to neurodegenerative illnesses such as Alzheimer's Disease and Lou Gehrig's Disease (ALS).

Some long-term studies show that regular consumption of artificially-sweetened beverages does reduce the intake of calories and can promote weight-loss or maintenance, but other research shows either no effect or even weight gain. A small number of studies show that artificial sweeteners can actually cause greater weight gain than regular sugar!

Studies also show that artificial sweeteners can:

- Increase hunger (!)
- Diminish insulin sensitivity to a greater degree than sugar.

(So if you're a diabetic, or diagnosed as pre-diabetic, it's best to stay away from all artificial sweeteners.)
- Cause many of the same illnesses associated with high sugar consumption (which include diabetes, stroke, and cardiovascular disease).

While you should eliminate all artificial sweeteners, there is one sugar alternative that can be used with caution:

Erythritol (a sugar alcohol)

Maybe it's because of the dangers found in artificial sweeteners that industry specialists have continued to try to find the perfect ingredient to keep your sweet tooth satisfied. And maybe that's why many "diet foods" now contain what are called sugar alcohols.

Sugar alcohols are refined, low-calorie, nutritive sweeteners. They are found naturally in the carbohydrates of many plants and fruits.

For instance,

Erythritol comes from corn or wheat starch.

Hydrogenated Starch Hydrolysate (HSH) comes from corn.

Isomalt comes from sucrose.

Lactitol comes from lactose.

Maltitol is an HSH created from corn syrup.

Mannitol comes from glucose syrup.

Sorbitol comes from glucose.

Xylitol comes traditionally from birch bark; today's sources are often made from corn.

Sugar alcohols are neither wholly sugar (they aren't metabolized in your body like sugar) nor wholly alcohol (they don't contain ethanol so they won't make you drunk). They're produced by using a chemical process that converts and then ferments (using bacteria or fungi) plant or fruit material. Even though chemically altered, sugar alcohols are still considered carbohydrates.

At the supermarket, you'll find sugar alcohols as the sweetening agents in "sugar-free" and "low-sugar" food products like chewing gum, candy, cookies, ice cream, soft drinks, and throat lozenges. They often show up in toothpaste and mouthwashes, too.

The reason they've become popular?
- They're used not only for their low-calorie sweet taste, but also because of their ability to preserve, add bulk, provide texture, retain moisture, and create cooling sensations in the mouth.
- Sugar alcohols won't cause tooth decay, and may even be able to fight bacterial growth. (For example, xylitol is currently being used to battle ear infections.)
- Sugar alcohols are considered diabetic-friendly. Certain sugar alcohols --- xylitol and mannitol, for instance --- are large molecules that don't break down entirely in your small intestine. Without being broken down, they can't be absorbed easily into your bloodstream. Instead, they'll pass through to your large intestine without spiking your blood sugar levels, and then be mostly eliminated in your urine.
- In contrast, sorbitol, maltitol, and isomalt are partially digested in the small intestine, can cause your blood levels to spike, and are not recommended for diabetics. (These are carbohydrates, after all.)

One reason that erythritol is singled out from other sugar alcohols as a sugar replacement is because of the way it responds in a person's digestive tract.

Because erythritol is a smaller molecule, it can be absorbed from the small intestine into the bloodstream and will eventually be excreted in the urine. But it's not broken down the way a normal sugar molecule is, and unlike sorbitol, maltitol, and isomalt, erythritol will not cause blood level spikes.

But here are the reasons why all sugar alcohols, including erythritol, should be used with caution:
1. If you eat a lot of them, you'll notice that you have to urinate more frequently. Increased urination, by the way,

means that you're probably also losing essential minerals like magnesium, potassium, and calcium --- the loss of which can cause cramping.

2. Sugar alcohols tend to ferment in the large intestine, causing gas, bloating, and diarrhea. (Because erythritol is partially broken down in the small intestine, it doesn't produce as much gas, bloating, or diarrhea as the others.)

3. All sugar alcohols are less sweet than sugar, containing somewhere from 30% to 90% of the sweetness, depending on which one we're talking about. (*Artificial* sweeteners, on the other hand, are usually 30-300 times sweeter than sugar.) But because sugar alcohols are less sweet than sugar, you typically have to use a larger amount to create the same sweetness level as sugar.

4. All sugar alcohols do have fewer calories than sugar --- but that doesn't mean that they're calorie-free. Most contain somewhere between 1.5 to 3 calories per gram, as compared to sugar's 4 calories per gram. For instance, xylitol contains 2.4 calories per gram, sorbitol 2.6 calories per gram, and hydrogenated starch (HSH) about 3 calories per gram.

5. Erythritol contains the least amount of calories, at 0.2 calories per gram. Extra caution here: Foods containing erythritol are often labeled "sugar-free" and "zero-calorie" even though erythritol does contain 0.2 calories per gram. While it's true that one serving adds up to a negligible amount of calories, if you eat enough of whatever the food is that contains erythritol, the calories will add up.

6. Sugar alcohols are refined products, and although found in nature, have been separated from their whole food sources and used as sweeteners for only a short time. (For example, erythritol was approved for use just as recently as 1990.) Not a lot of research has been done to note the effect these refined products have on humans. All refined

products are able to affect a human body more quickly and intensely than a non-refined product.

7. Sugar alcohols are considered low-glycemic and low-calorie because they are only partially digested and partially absorbed in the upper gastrointestinal tract. Nevertheless, before being eliminated in your urine and while they are still in the large intestine, they are known to ferment, causing gas, bloating, and diarrhea. (Erythritol does not seem to create the same amount of gastric distress as other sugar alcohols, and for this reason might be the best choice among all sugar alcohols.) Sarah Pope, author of The Healthy Home Economist website, notes that consuming highly refined products like sugar alcohols opens the door to creating or contributing to gut imbalance. And gut imbalance is not what you want if you want to be healthy! You want a properly functioning digestive system with a harmoniously settled gut biome.

8. *Sugar alcohols are often combined with artificial sweeteners to reach the required sweetness level food producers desire, and consumers seem to want. They are also commonly found in foods that have other questionable ingredients like refined carbohydrates and chemically processed oils.*

9. If one of the reasons you're with me right now is to free yourself from sugar addiction, you've got to consider all the ways that can help you be free. By continuing to use artificial and low-calorie sweeteners, your taste buds never get a chance to "understand" what natural sweetness is.

10. If you substitute *artificial sweeteners* for sugar, you're training your taste buds to stay addicted to the sweet taste of sugar. With each serving of artificial sweeteners, you condition yourself to need sweeter and sweeter foods to be satisfied.

11. If you substitute *low-calorie sweeteners* for sugar, you're tempted to overeat foods that contain them because your mind is telling you: "It's okay because there's no sugar inside."

12. The American Diabetes Association contends that sugar alcohols are acceptable in moderate amounts, but it does warn that you should not eat them in excess. They've noted that some people with diabetes, especially Type I Diabetes, have found that their blood sugars rise if sugar alcohols are eaten in unlimited amounts.

13. SIBO (small intestinal bacterial overgrowth) can be exacerbated with the use of sugar alcohols. Beneficial bacteria are necessary for your body to be able to absorb nutrients and to maintain healthy bowel movements. Too many sugar alcohols can cause toxic bacteria to proliferate. With too much toxic bacteria, you won't be absorbing the nutrients you need or eliminating the waste your digestive system must remove in order for you to remain healthy.

While you should eliminate all artificial sweeteners, **three sugar alternatives can be used in moderation:**

1. **Stevia**: is considered a natural, zero-calorie sweetener that's extracted from the leaf of the South American stevia plant. The leaf contains two sweet compounds: stevioside and rebaudioside A. Stevioside appears to have some health benefits --- like lowering blood sugar levels and reducing blood pressure --- but rebaudioside A does not. Stevia is 300 times as sweet as sugar, and because of this is often sold with a bulking agent like dextrose or erythritol. Reading the packaging label --- both front and back --- is important. Beware of the particular brand known as Stevia in The Raw. The first ingredient listed is dextrose (another word for glucose and made from corn --- often GMO corn), and dextrose could make up 90% of the packet, meaning that the health benefits of stevia would be minimal, and each

teaspoon-serving would contain about 15 calories!

Truvia (a brand-name Stevia product) is not considered a safe alternative (at least science can't confirm that it is). Presently Truvia is manufactured using only the part of the stevia plant --- Rebaudioside A --- that provides most of the sweet taste.

Coca-Cola and Cargill (a food additive manufacturer) developed Truvia combining three main ingredients: erythritol, Rebaudioside A, and "natural flavors." Stevioside (the part of the stevia leaf with the health-giving benefits) is not included. Erythritol is a sugar alcohol that can pass through your system and out of your body without any of the harmful effects of sugar. So in this sense, Truvia could be considered harmless (except for some it may cause digestive distress).

But Cargill, who manufactures Truvia, will not disclose what specific substances make up its "natural flavors." Remember that hydrolyzed vegetable protein (MSG) can legally be listed on a label as a "natural flavor." Without knowing all of Truvia's ingredients, who can say for sure if it's safe?

2. **Lo Han Guo**: also known as *monk fruit*. Grown mostly in China, this fruit is a type of gourd whose flesh is 200 times sweeter than sugar. The fruit is used only after it is dried, and can be processed into a powder that contains natural substances called *mogrosides*. The curious thing about these mogrosides is that they have been shown to regulate blood sugar levels. The fruit contains a large amount of glucose but only about 13% fructose.

3. **Glucose**: an expensive alternative to sugar.
Dr. Mercola writes that pure glucose is a healthy, natural alternative to sugar (sucrose) for your sweet tooth. Because it is only 70 percent as sweet as sucrose, Dr. Mercola suggests that you might end up using a bit more of it for the same amount of sweetness. Using more might make it slightly more expensive than regular sugar, but the price could still be well worth it for your health since glucose doesn't contain any fructose in its composition.

By now all of this information may have unsettled you. You're wondering if there's *anything else* besides scandalous sugar, alarming artificial sweeteners, chemically extracted sugar alcohols, or other sugar alternatives *that you can regularly use* to flavor your water *without* sacrificing your health.

Is there anything that can add some variation to your water without causing you to gain weight?

Is there anything to add to your water that can actually help you lose weight?

Yes! And it's been kept a secret for way too long.

There *is* one sugar alternative that you can add to your water which will not cause you to gain weight and can actually help you lose weight: Apple Cider Vinegar.

Apple Cider Vinegar: Weight-Loss Secret #3A
Taking Apple Cider Vinegar Before A Meal Can Help You Lose Weight. (Most secrets are discovered by accident, and this one was, too.)

In 2004 an associate director of the School of Nutrition and Health Promotion at Arizona State University named Dr. Carol S. Johnston was testing a theory which said: vinegar can reduce cholesterol levels.

While that didn't produce positive results at the time (a later study in 2006, conducted on rats, showed vinegar to lower cholesterol), Professor Johnston discovered something else: that participants who took 2 tablespoons of apple cider vinegar (mixed in 8 ounces of water) before their lunch and dinner meals lost an average of 2 pounds during her 4-week trial. (The odd thing noted by Dr. Johnston was that this study was performed during the holiday season when people tend to eat more than usual!) "Acetic acid, the main component in vinegar, may interfere with the body's ability to digest starch... If you're interfering with the digestion of starch, less is broken down into calories in the bloodstream. Over time, that might cause a subtle effect on weight," Professor Johnston explained.

A later Dutch study in 2012 did find that in one North African culture, women who consumed a daily cup of apple cider vinegar achieved greater weight-loss than women who did not.

Apple Cider Vinegar: Weight-Loss Secret #3B

- *Taking Apple Cider Vinegar Before a Meal Can Help Satisfy Your Appetite.*

  Maybe Dr. Johnston's study showed the 2-pound loss because of another one of the "by-products" of apple cider vinegar: its effectiveness in reducing appetite. During the year following Dr. Johnston's study, researchers at Lund University in Sweden tested apple cider vinegar's effect on insulin production and glucose levels after eating. These same studies also examined satiety: were the subjects less hungry shortly after eating if they had taken vinegar before their meals? And you already know the answer: they were!

Apple Cider Vinegar's Well-kept Weight-Loss Secret #3C

- *Taking Apple Cider Vinegar Before a Meal Can Burn Fat.*

  The breakthrough study for showing vinegar as a successful tool for burning fat didn't come until July 2009, when Japanese researchers conducted a study using a high-fat diet on laboratory mice. Mice that were given vinegar in addition to their regular menu developed less body fat than mice whose food did not include vinegar.

  Why does it work?

  While the fat-burning qualities of vinegar are still a bit unclear, both Johnston and Tomoo Kondo, who performed the 2009 study, believe that the acetic acid in vinegar is the reason it works. Essentially, the acetic acid leads to the body's production of proteins that will break down the fat and help prevent build-up in the body.

As long as you don't have a problem tolerating high-acid foods, drinking apple cider vinegar won't hurt you, says Kimberly Gomer, a registered dietitian at the Pritikin Longevity Center + Spa in Miami.

But don't consume too much; undiluted apple cider vinegar will burn your throat and eat away at your tooth enamel. All vinegars contain acetic acid, but the safe ones for consumption have no more than 5% acidity, and this amount should be written on the label.

The best kind to use is raw, organic, apple cider vinegar with the "mother" still intact. (Apple cider vinegar with the mother is merely unrefined, unpasteurized, and unfiltered apple cider vinegar that looks cloudy, not clear. The mother is a collection of fiber-strands made up of yeast and acetic acid bacteria, formed from naturally occurring pectin and apple residues. The presence of the mother is evidence that the valuable, health-giving components of the apple haven't been destroyed. Vinegars with the mother contain enzymes and minerals that are missing from other vinegars because of over-processing, filtration, and overheating.)

One added benefit of Apple Cider Vinegar: Weight-Loss Secret #3D

- Many people carry around a few (10? 20?) extra pounds merely because they're not digesting their food!
  So, if you have digestive problems, apple cider vinegar may be just the solution for you. *Apple cider vinegar stimulates digestive juices which help your body break down food, reduce gas, and relieve constipation.*

Today's Goals:

Eliminate all artificial sweeteners from your diet.

Use low-calorie sweeteners with caution.

Use natural sweeteners in moderation.

Enjoy the benefits of apple cider vinegar!

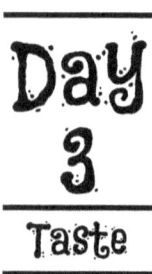

Day 3
Taste

TANGY APPLE CIDER VINEGAR DRINK
(Serves 1)

Ingredients:

12 ounces chilled, purified, or spring water
1 tablespoon apple cider vinegar *(unrefined, unfiltered, unpasteurized)*
1 teaspoon Manuka honey *(or raw, unrefined, local honey)*

Directions:

- Pour water into a tall glass.
- Add in the apple cider vinegar.
- Add in the Manuka honey. *(If the honey is too dense to dissolve easily, first warm the jar under hot water before extracting a teaspoon of it.)*
- Mix all ingredients together.
- Drink and enjoy!

Day 3
move

SIT...

while eating.

(But don't eat while driving.)

Plan to have each meal --- not on the run --- but at a time and place where you can sit down and not have to rush.

If you don't have time to sit down, then wait to eat.

Sitting will help to relax you, calm you, and calm your autonomic nervous system --- that automatic mechanism which controls bodily functions without your having to think about them.

Digestion is part of your autonomic nervous system. You don't have to tell it how to do its job, but you can interfere with its efficiency if you eat while standing, walking or driving, or have stressful conversations even while sitting. Allowing your body to break down and absorb the food you eat without hindrances is so very important for your health and well-being.

Sitting calmly helps your digestive tract do its work without stress or distraction or energy spent elsewhere.

Help it out.

Drink a glass of water about twenty minutes before you eat.

Breathe before you eat.

Sit down to eat.

And enjoy the gift of food.

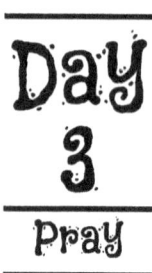

THE SWEET BEAUTY OF SELF-CONTROL

Hello God,

You provided honey for its sweetness,

but you also offered advice that I shouldn't eat too much of it.

Which means that I have the power to control how many desserts I have.

Or if I'm not experiencing that power now, you can help me gain back that control.

Let me know how.

You want me to be a strong city, well-defended against outside attacks.

Help me begin to practice self-control and build my city walls one brick at a time.

There is beauty in self-control.

Help me to be handsome or beautiful on the inside --- the part of me that really matters to you.

Help me to resist sweets as I resist seeking my own honor.

Proverbs 25:27-28

*It is not good to eat too much honey,
nor is it honorable to seek one's own honor.
Like a city whose walls are broken through
is a person who lacks self-control.*

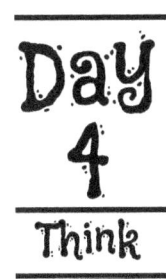

SPICING UP WATER...WITH TEA!

Good morning.

Welcome to Day 4, and come on into the kitchen so I can fix you a nice cup of tea.

Oh so many choices we have to dress up your water. Would you like it hot or cold? Herbal or caffeinated?

Since you're on a search to lose weight, maintain a healthy weight, or increase your energy, I'm first going to recommend an herbal tea, especially if you have difficulty with caffeine. (You might want to know, though, that caffeine --- because of its stimulating effect --- has been shown in numerous studies to improve exercise performance and aid fat burning!)

Drinking teas while you're trying to lose weight is a good practice because most teas contain almost no calories. They can help you feel satisfied and full without adding empty calories and/or toxic substances that sugared sodas or juices contain.

One herbal tea you may not have thought of: dandelion root tea.

Drinking dandelion root tea, especially before meals, or even in soups or juices, may enhance your weight-loss because of the way dandelion root stimulates gastric secretions. These secretions breakdown fats and cholesterol, helping your body excrete them before they are absorbed.

Caution:
According to the University of Maryland Medical Center, dandelion leaves act as a diuretic. So if you include large quantities of dandelion

leaf tea during the next 21 days, you could end up losing not just body fat, but a large amount of water weight as well. Check to see if you're losing more than 2 to 3 pounds weekly. If so, chances are that some of what you're shedding is water weight. While water weight-loss is tolerable if you're holding excess fluid, too much water loss can cause dehydration. Please cut back on dandelion leaf tea if you experience any symptoms of dehydration.

Is dandelion tea safe in all cases?
The University of Maryland Medical Center reports that dandelion is generally safe, but it may trigger allergic reactions in some people and can interact with certain medications, supplements, and other herbs. The center suggests using caution when ingesting dandelion with antacids, diuretics, diabetes medications, or blood-thinning medications.

An Alternative to Dandelion Tea

On the other hand, if your system has some tolerance for caffeine, you can choose green, white or oolong tea for effective use in weight-loss. (The truth is, decaffeinated teas or herbal teas are less effective teas for weight-loss.) Of course, choosing sweetened teas or diet teas would be entirely counterproductive.

Weight-Loss Secrets in Matcha Green Tea

Matcha tea is not an herbal tea in regards to caffeine. Matcha is a green tea that contains caffeine, but each cup contains much less than a cup of coffee, and this tea is very much worth including in your diet.

Did you know there is magic in the leaves?

Matcha tea hasn't been called "the elixir of the immortals" for nothing. Studies have shown that not only does it benefit your heart, your liver, your joints, your hair, and your skin...but it also fights cancer.

Okay, okay. I know we're here to talk about how matcha green tea can help you lose weight and give you energy, but ---

I want to emphasize:
When you increase your liquid intake by sipping on a magic

potion of matcha green tea (or *Camellia Sinensis*), you will not only be losing weight enjoyably, but you'll be increasing the health of your whole body.

"Matcha" means powdered, and the manufacturing of this green tea involves a process that grinds the whole green tea leaf into powder. So when you drink matcha green tea, you're actually consuming every single part of the green tea leaf, not just steeping a green leaf in boiling water. This is a critical detail to understand because drinking regular green tea will not give you all of the benefits of losing weight that you are looking for.

How does matcha green tea help you lose weight?

In 6 specific ways.

1. **Matcha boosts your fat metabolism.**

    Thermogenesis is the process of heat production in organisms. When heat production is raised, more energy is used. When more energy is used, more calories are burned.

    Lucky for you that matcha tea has been shown to increase thermogenesis in the human body, and its thermogenic properties and ability to oxidize fat go beyond what caffeine can account for.

2. **Matcha can prevent an increase in fat tissue…**
    because of the following components it contains:

    - *Theanine*, an amino acid which can naturally calm and focus your brain.

    People generally use theanine for treating anxiety or stress as well as high blood pressure. But what is helpful for you to know is that there's a huge relationship between stress and obesity. Did you know that stress hormones (like cortisol and adrenaline) cause a person's fat tissue to increase?

    When you drink matcha tea, however, the theanine in it will induce a state of relaxation in your brain. By calming your mind with matcha, your body, through its sympathetic nervous system, will not be "commanded" to hoard extra fat around your waist and organs.

- *Green tea catechins*, which are a type of flavonoid having many health benefits. Epigallocatechin gallate (EGCG), present in green tea, is the catechin responsible for heightened weight-loss. EGCG promotes weight-loss by boosting your metabolism and --- because of its effect on fat-burning hormones --- promotes fat breakdown. Green tea catechins especially attack the fat in your abdominal area. (Studies show that while green tea catechins seem to be effective at promoting weight-loss, the catechins found in other foods don't seem to have the same effect.)

3. **Matcha can suppress your appetite.**
   This happens through the following specific components matcha tea contains:

   - *Soluble fiber*, which helps to pass food through your digestive tract.

   - *Caffeine*, which is able to stimulate your central nervous system, increase your heart and respiration rates, and can act as a gentle diuretic.

   - *The combination of soluble fiber, caffeine, theanine, and green tea catechins.* It turns out that it's the combination of these ingredients which is probably responsible for decreased carbohydrate and sugar cravings.

4. **Matcha reduces inflammation.**
   Chronic inflammation is now being shown to be the hidden cause of many illnesses, and current studies are specifically demonstrating the relationship between chronic inflammation and obesity. So reducing inflammation can actually help you lose weight.

   Polyphenols are plant nutrients that have been shown to fight inflammation, and polyphenols (in the form on EGCGs), are exceptionally plentiful in matcha green tea.

5. **Matcha purifies and cleanses.**
   Matcha helps to pull toxins out of your cells, into your

bloodstream, and then filters them out of your body. A recent study showed that rats who ate food laced with toxic chemicals along with matcha green tea excreted 4x the poison than the control group.

Studies also reveal that when poisons which have been stored in the fat cells of the human body are released, more fat cells are released along with them!

Matcha's cleansing power is probably due to the chlorophyll it contains. When chlorophyll is introduced into your blood and body tissues, it first neutralizes your whole system from becoming too acidic. Then, as the chlorophyll moves along your digestive tract, it brushes harmful toxins from the walls of your large intestine (where waste accumulates) and ultimately helps carry the acidic residue with it right out of your body. Getting rid of waste, it turns out, is extra-important for not only releasing your body of its extra weight, but also for regulating your mood so you maintain the desire to continue on with your goals.

6. **Matcha can kill *Candida albicans*.**
Candida is a fungus (or a form of yeast) that often lives undetected in the bodies of most people. When uncontrolled, *Candida* causes a vast array of problems. Oral thrush, constant vaginal infections, athlete's foot, nail fungus, bloating, constipation, diarrhea, and chronic fatigue are some symptoms of *Candida albicans* gone wild.

Candida can also obstruct your ability to lose weight. How? It cranks up your sugar cravings, causes bloating and turns your mood downward. Do you find yourself always yearning for sugary donuts, cookies, cakes, or fast food? You might have a *Candida* problem. And matcha tea would be a good solution for you because of its ability to help kill *Candida albicans*, as well as other yeasts. Plus, it creates a favorable environment for good bacteria to grow. And good bacteria in your system is necessary for proper digestion.

Here are some things to consider as you incorporate theanine and green tea catechins into your daily schedule:

The most natural and easiest way to get them into your diet is to drink regular green tea.

A daily dose of 270 mg of catechins is the amount an average person would need to achieve maximum benefits for weight-loss. (This is according to a study published in the December 1999 issue of The American Journal of Clinical Nutrition.)

The average cup of freshly brewed loose leaf green tea (not matcha) has about 50-70 mg of EGCG (otherwise known as epigallocatechin gallate, or the green tea catechin most responsible for weight-loss) in it --- which would mean drinking 3 to 5 cups of double-brewed green tea each day to achieve maximum benefits. (Freshly brewed green tea contains more than decaffeinated, instant, or pre-made teas.)

Matcha is ten times more potent than regular green tea. One teaspoon (the amount you might mix into one cup --- or 12 ounces of liquid) contains about 120 mg of EGCG.

Two cups a day would set you up for effective weight-loss and a healthy weight.

Catechin extract supplements are all different, so it's necessary to pay attention to the ingredients. Speak to your doctor about safety if things like yohimbe, willow bark extract, or additional theobromine are added to the supplement.

You should also prepare your teas with low-protein liquids like water, coconut milk, or almond milk. Cow's milk is heavy in protein and not a good choice for matcha.

Today's Goal:

Have a cup of green tea. (Check *www.kriswilliamswellness.com* for excellent sources of green tea and matcha tea.)

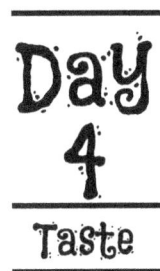

MATCHA TEA SPECIAL
(Serves 1)

Ingredients:

6 ounces almond milk *(unsweetened, plain or vanilla)*
6 ounces purified or spring water
½ to 1 teaspoon pure matcha tea *(or 2 teaspoons of matcha chai for an added thrill!)*
stevia to taste

Directions:

- Pour the almond milk & water into a heavy saucepan.
- Add the matcha tea to the liquid.
- Sprinkle in a dash of stevia.
- Whisk all ingredients together, then bring to a boil.
- Pour into a cup.
- Let cool slightly --- then ---
- Drink and enjoy! *(Believe me, you will!)*

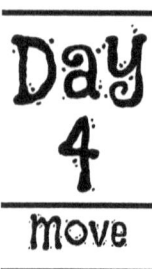

CHEW WELL

Chew well each bite of food you put into your mouth.

If food is served to you in pieces larger than the size of what would fit on a teaspoon or fork, then cut what is in front of you into pieces that *will* fit.

Deposit each portion into your mouth and ---

Chew --- at least 10 or 15 times!

If this sounds ridiculous, remember that I promised you some humor.

And also remember that: digestion begins in the mouth.

Have you ever tried to chew your food 20 times, which is what nutritionists recommend?

I'm suggesting 5 fewer chews.

Because 15 chews will allow you to really taste what you're eating.

(And if you're like me, and I know I am, you've previously gulped down food that you've barely tasted --- because you failed to chew it.)

So today, at each meal, cut your food, and chew each bite 15 times.

Humor me?

Eat to enjoy the good gifts given to you by the One who made them for your enjoyment.

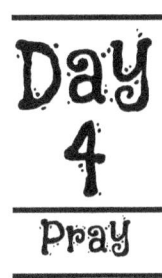

I WANT TO THANK YOU

Hello God,

Will you help me to pause before I eat,

each and every time,

in order to thank you for the food that is before me?

Will you remind me to thank you for the farmers who grew it, the workers who harvested it, and the animals who gave their lives to provide it?

I recognize that there are people all over the world who don't have enough of what I have in abundance.

I know that it will take a little bit of time --- and thought --- to thank you for farmers and workers and animals.

So, will you help me to understand that these few moments of thanks before a meal or a snack are meant to help me eat mindfully?

Will you show me that these few moments of thanks will help me to eat taste-fully?

Will you show me that these few moments of thanks will help me to eat without rushing?

Will you show me that these few moments of thanks will help me appreciate the good gifts you provide?

Psalm 107:8-9

*Let them give thanks to the LORD
for his unfailing love
and his wonderful deeds for mankind,
for he satisfies the thirsty
and fills the hungry with good things.*

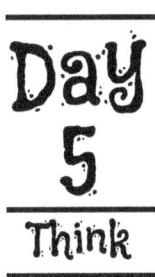

Day 5
Think

SURPRISED BY WHAT YOU'RE FULL OF?

Day 5 is upon us, you're visiting me, sipping tea, and wondering why I'm talking about bacteria.

Is your body really full of it?

Yes, but being full of it is not all bad.

Somewhere around 100 trillion bacteria camp out in your body every day. And about 1 quadrillion (or 1,000 trillion) viruses --- called bacteriophages --- join them.

The truth is that every single person is like a moving city filled with what could be hazardous microscopic organisms. The bacteria that live in your body actually outnumber the rest of your cells 10 to 1. The bacteriophages, in turn, outnumber bacteria 10 to 1.

Added to bacteria and bacteriophages are fungi (or yeasts --- such as *Candida albicans*) that are present in many people and in varying amounts.

Makes you just want to drink Lysol, right?

Nevertheless, all of these organisms --- the bacteria, the bacteriophages, and the yeasts --- are necessary for your body because they help with: assimilating and digesting the food you eat; producing vitamin B-12, butyrate, and vitamin K2; creating enzymes that destroy harmful bacteria; stimulating secretion of IgA and regulatory T Cells... In other words, they work in many body processes to keep you balanced and healthy (both mentally and physically), aid in weight-loss, and promote maintaining a proper weight.

The problems come when bad bacteria move into certain neighborhoods of your "city." It's when harmful bacteria and yeast proliferate --- when they grow to outnumber the beneficial bacteria --- that you experience inflammation and a whole list of illnesses that disturb your mind, break down your body, prevent you from losing weight, and even cause you to gain weight!

Want to know what kills good bacteria?

Leading the list are the following surprising (or not so surprising) substances:

- Prescription antibiotics (these are drugs that kill *all* of your bacteria..good *and* bad)
- Sugar
- Unfiltered tap water
- GMO foods
- Grains
- Emotional stress
- Chemicals and other prescription medications

One of the first real studies to reveal that flora in your digestive tract (or gut bacteria) affect how much you weigh was conducted at the Washington University School of Medicine in St. Louis in 2006. Researchers there found that obese people had different gut bacteria than normal-weighted people.

Later studies revealed that gut neighborhoods in lean people were full of a variety of beneficial bacteria, but in obese people, there was much less diversity, and much less of the good bacteria. Lean participants in the study tended to have a wider variety of microbes called *Bacteroidetes*, which are useful in breaking down thick plant starches and fibers so that the resulting substances can be used for energy.

But even before 2006, results from a study in 2004 headed by Professor Angelo Tremblay at the Université Laval in Canada provided much encouragement and hope. Tremblay and his researchers discovered that good bacteria could promote weight-loss! This old news should make you happy, too!

The study was conducted in this way:

Good bacteria (the kind that aids in food digestion, not the kind that promotes disease) were introduced into the digestive tracts of 125 people.

After the study's initial 12-week dieting period, the research team observed an average weight-loss of about 10 pounds (4.4 kg) in women who were consuming the "right bacteria." (Curiously, no differences in weight-loss were observed among males, and the researchers weren't sure whether it was a question of dosage, or just because the study was too short. More research is needed here.)

One of the impressive things about this study for women is that after the end of another 12 weeks without dieting (called the maintenance period), the women taking the right bacteria continued to drop their weight, losing an average of 11.5 pounds (5.2kg) per person.

With testing, it was discovered that these women had a more active appetite-regulating hormone, as well as less of the intestinal bacteria related to obesity.

So what are these fantastic "good" bacteria called, why do they work, and where can you get them?

Good bacteria (and yeast) that are strong enough to fight the bad are known as *probiotics*.

In his book, *Probiotics For Dummies (2012)*, Dr. Shekhar K. Challa, a gastroenterologist, explains that probiotics do their work by "crowding out" bad bacteria. There are only so many places along your intestinal walls that bacteria can "latch" onto. If good bacteria take up all --- or most of --- the spots, then there are fewer --- or no --- "latches" available for the bad bacteria.

Because bacteria in the intestinal tract participate in the processes of breaking down food and absorbing nutrients, it's essential to have good bacteria available to do this important work. Otherwise, food isn't broken down thoroughly, and nutrients aren't absorbed properly.

An alarming side-fact gleaned from this and additional studies was that the bacteria in overweight humans actually absorb more calories from food than the bacteria in thin people. From his research in 2004, Dr. Tremblay also concluded that bad bacteria may make the intestinal wall more permeable, and the badly metabolized calories then end up in fat cells. Probiotics make your intestinal walls stronger and more able to prevent poorly digested foods and their byproducts (which cause inflammation) from passing through the intestines and into the bloodstream.

Another reason why it's vital to maintain the health of your gut is because you have a second brain living there!

All along your alimentary canal (food passageway) are 100 million neurons which make up this second brain. These nerve fibers are able to make digestion "decisions" on their own, and they also communicate other functional information back to the brain in your head. Your second brain plays a big part in your emotional state. If it is overcome by unhealthy, bad bacteria, you may feel extremely moody or "out of control." Your emotional well-being relies on your lower brain to send the correct, unhindered messages to your upper brain. An alimentary canal filled with bad bacteria will text all the wrong messages that could end up sinking you into a sour mood, plunging you into a depressed state, or stealing away your energy. To keep yourself committed to your health and weight-loss goals, it's necessary for your gut to produce good bacteria.

How can you enhance the production of good bacteria --- or probiotics --- in your system?

Start by eating plenty of *prebiotics* --- fibrous carbohydrates such as broccoli, celery, carrots, Brussel sprouts --- that require some work for your system to digest. Beneficial bacteria thrive on these fibrous or hard-to-digest carbohydrates. Fiber-rich fruits and vegetables, as well as onions, artichokes, whole grains, and garlic in particular, can stimulate the growth of good gut flora, also.

Probiotics (which can include strains of bacteria as well as certain types of yeasts) can be found in certain fermented foods or drink. Fermented foods include things like: sauerkraut, plain unflavored yogurt, miso, kimchi, pickles, tempeh, kombucha tea, kefir, certain surprising foods some people crave (like dark chocolate!) and certain supplements you can choose to take. If you're not partial to sauerkraut, yogurt,* miso, kimchi, or kefir, then taking probiotics in supplement form might be the best alternative.**

Besides fighting obesity, with probiotics you'll also be fighting infections, boosting your immune system, reducing inflammation, and improving your overall health!

***Beware of commercial yogurts for 2 reasons:**
- They often contain large amounts of added sugar.
- They often have most of their beneficial bacteria processed out of them due to the high temperatures used in pasteurization.
  Some manufacturers add probiotics after the yogurt has been treated with heat, so if you can verify that this has been done, you should be confident you're actually receiving the advantages of probiotics when you eat this yogurt.

**The best way to include probiotics is by eating fermented foods.

Today's Goal:

Determine which way is the easiest way for you to take in probiotics: in food form or as a supplement.

Check *www.kriswilliamswellness.com* for sauerkraut and kefir sources, as well as for good sources of probiotic supplements.

Most people experience transforming results by including a daily probiotic that contains at least 50 billion CFUs (colony-forming units).

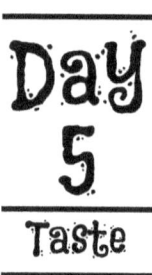

Day 5
Taste

RAW SAUERKRAUT
(makes about 1/2 quart)

Ingredients:

1 quart Mason jar
1/2 medium head of unwashed organic cabbage *(green, purple, napa, or combination of all three)*
2 tablespoons pink Himalayan salt (test amount for taste)

Directions:
- Chop or shred cabbage, leaving root end attached. Sprinkle with salt.
- Knead cabbage with clean hands, or pound with a potato masher or cabbage crusher for about 10 minutes --- (until there is enough liquid to cover it when you place it in the jar.)
- Stuff the cabbage into the jar *(it should fill to about half-way up)*, add the liquid & press the cabbage underneath the liquid.
- Use reserved leaves to help weigh down the chopped cabbage. *(You may need to add a bit of water to completely cover the chopped cabbage.)*
- Cover the jar with a coffee filter or cheesecloth & secure with a rubber band. *(If using a tight lid instead of a coffee filter or cheesecloth, "burp" the jar daily to release excess pressure. Do this by unscrewing the lid and letting the gas out!)*
- Let sit at room temperature (65-72°F) for 3-7 days.
- Once the sauerkraut is ready *("readiness" is according to your taste; longer aging increases the flavor)*, secure a tight lid on the jar & move it to your refrigerator. *(This stores for about 2 weeks.)*
- Enjoy!

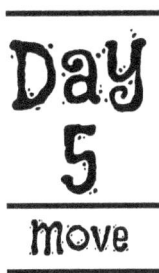

Day 5
move

SIT UP STRAIGHT

Sit up straight while eating ---

And ---

Sit up straight while working at a desk or computer.

It's easy to slouch.

When you slouch, your organs fold in on themselves, and your back muscles weaken.

To sit up straight:

Move forward in your chair so that your feet can be placed flat on the floor.

With your feet flat on the floor, rotate your hips forward.

With your hips rotated forward, your stomach will "open-up," and your shoulders will rotate back naturally.

Sitting with your hips rotated forward, back straight, and shoulders unrounded will prevent neck strain and a sore back.

Sitting this way will energize you and build strong back muscles.

Be energized!

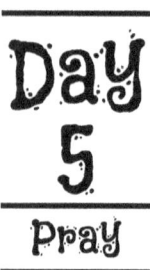

Day 5
Pray

ONE GOOD HABIT WILL MAKE ME STRONGER

Hello, God,

My body is so much more amazing than I ever realized.

Not only did you design millions of separate parts for it, but you also made sure that all of the parts would work together for my good.

It's too big of a design for me to fathom!

And who knew that I have not just one brain, but two!

A brain in my gut!

A thing like that!

Thanks for letting me know today how important it is to feed this second brain the right kind of nutrients. I never knew how much the health of this gut-brain affects the amount of weight I gain or lose. I never realized how much this second brain affects my moods.

But I *have* noticed how much my moods affect other parts of my life.

My moods can disrupt how I sleep, causing me to be up at 3am, anxious or restless.

My moods can affect how well I work, making me feel justified in not following through with one commitment or another because I "don't feel up to it."

Sour moods affect how I think, causing a lot of negative self-talk.

Moodiness can control the way I communicate with other people, causing me to become impatient, unnecessarily aggressive, to snap at people, or to want to repeatedly withdraw from everyone. Moodiness given in to can leave me very depressed.

And I can go for days being pulled and tossed like an emotional yo-yo.

Moodiness can even destroy my dreams and goals for exercising, eating healthfully, and completing the work you have for me to do. I lose the energy and desire to continue.

I confess that my moods control me a lot.

Moodiness makes me feel like I have no self-discipline.

I hate it when I have no self-discipline.

And I want to confess this to you. And to ask you to forgive me for the times I am impatient, aggressive, snappy, or lacking self-discipline.

So I am finally at the place where I know I need to ask you:

Will you train me in your discipline?

And if controlling my gut biome will really help, will you show me all the ways I can restore health to this second brain by making sure it gets all the prebiotics and probiotics it needs?

I Corinthians 9: 25-27

Everyone who competes in the games goes into strict training.
They do it to get a crown that will not last,
but we do it to get a crown that will last forever.
Therefore I do not run like someone running aimlessly;
I do not fight like a boxer beating the air.
No, I strike a blow to my body and make it my slave
so that after I have preached to others,
I myself will not be disqualified for the prize.

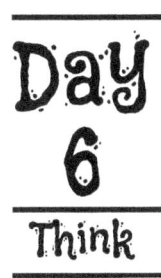

Day 6
Think

WHAT'S MAGNESIUM GOT TO DO WITH IT?

In her book *The Magnesium Miracle (2003)*, Carolyn Dean, M.D., N.D., states three causes for gaining weight around your middle:

1. A magnesium deficiency
2. Your body's inability to digest, absorb, and utilize proteins, fats, and carbohydrates. (Magnesium is essential for the function of these processes.)
3. The abundance of obesity genes "expressing themselves." (Every person is born with a complete set of DNA --- or a complete set of genes containing all the information needed to build and maintain that person's life. It is possible that certain people are born with obesity genes in their DNA; these people become obese if these genes are allowed to operate freely or "express themselves." Magnesium, it turns out, can help prevent obesity genes from expressing themselves.)

With this information, it seems like a good idea to be well-supplied with magnesium!

But most people in the modern world are...magnesium-deficient.

Could you be one of them?

How does a magnesium deficiency happen?
- It happens when a person fails to eat a variety of foods like whole grains, vegetables, legumes, nuts, and seeds. The best sources of magnesium are whole, organic foods --- especially dark green leafy vegetables. Other good sources

include seaweed, dried pumpkin seeds, unsweetened cocoa, flaxseed, almond butter, and whey.

- It happens when a person eats foods that are highly-processed. Fast-food restaurants and grocery stores sell foods that are highly-refined, heavily preserved foods that probably have magnesium processed right out of them. So if fast-foods and packaged-foods make up a good portion of your diet, then you, too, are probably magnesium-deficient.

- It happens because people live in a modern world. Modern farming practices have depleted magnesium and other vital minerals from large portions of America's growing soil. If the soil in which whole grains, green leafy vegetables, beans, nuts, and seeds grow is low in magnesium, then the whole grains, green leafy vegetables, legumes, nuts, and seeds produced will be low in magnesium, as well.

- It happens because medications (including common diuretics, birth control pills, insulin, some antibiotics, and cortisone) cause the body to use up or deplete a person's magnesium supply.

- It happens because taking antacids (and some other medicines for indigestion) disrupts magnesium absorption.

Why does magnesium have a starring role in weight-loss?

When you eat, magnesium activates hundreds of enzymes in your body --- including digestive enzymes --- so you can process every morsel of food that goes into your mouth. Without magnesium --- without this "tool" that facilitates the breakdown and absorption of the fats, proteins, and carbohydrates you eat every day --- your body doesn't get all the nutrients it requires. Without all the critical nutrients your body needs, you end up hankering to eat more…and more…in an effort to obtain those vital nutrients.

When you are between meals, magnesium in your system helps to keep your hunger cravings in check.

If there's not enough magnesium in your system, your bowel movements can slow down or stop, food putrefies in your digestive tract, your gut protrudes, and you end up distressed and sick as a result. As you may have already experienced, a distressed and sick body will not work to lose weight.

Magnesium influences insulin, the hormone you first heard about on Day 2. Insulin is a dominant factor in weight control because it helps regulate blood sugar. Some people have high levels of insulin in their blood either because they eat too much sugar or highly processed foods, or because their bodies fail to use insulin effectively. And since insulin causes fat to be stored in fat cells, high levels of insulin cause lots of fat to be stored in lots of fat cells.

When your body continues to fail to use insulin effectively, you're known as being insulin resistant, and when you're insulin resistant, your blood sugar levels continue to increase. Magnesium helps insulin do its job more effectively and keeps your blood levels in check.

Magnesium seems to be the number one mineral for improving insulin sensitivity. On the other hand, magnesium deficiency has been found to cause insulin resistance --- which leads to hyperinsulinemia, then hypertension, then diabetes, then...

There's more to weight-loss than counting calories or using willpower to resist high-calorie foods, sweets, or extra servings.

On Day 2 you also heard about leptin, that hormone stimulated by insulin which triggers your sense of feeling full. If leptin is allowed to communicate freely with your brain, you'll feel satisfied with normal servings of food, and shouldn't be led to overeat. Magnesium is a mineral that increases your brain's sensitivity to leptin.

Magnesium also helps you get a better night's sleep. Dr. Mark Hyman labeled magnesium "the most powerful relaxation mineral available" because of its calming effect on your body's nervous system and its relaxing effect on your muscles. Sleep is made possible with calm nerves and relaxed muscles. Magnesium may also improve the length and quality of slow-wave sleep, also known as "good sleep." And good sleep is primary if you want to lose weight, maintain a healthy weight, or gain back the energy you need. Sleep for your body is like the "off-switch" for your computer. Using the off-switch for your computer allows the whole mechanism to be reset and rebooted. Adequate sleep for you means allowing your body a chance to reboot. When you regularly permit yourself to sleep long enough and deeply enough, you give your body a fighting chance to restore itself. If you don't get enough deep sleep, you may be prone to overeat because your body is trying to take in the energy that you should have naturally stored up from your night-time rest.

Stress is a significant factor that inhibits your ability to lose weight, too.

Here's how it happens:

- Stress triggers your adrenal glands to secrete a hormone called *cortisol*.
- Cortisol triggers the flight or fight response.
- Over time an oversupply of cortisol diminishes the power of your thyroid glands --- glands which produce hormones that are responsible for regulating your metabolism.
- If your metabolism isn't adequately regulated, your body stops breaking down food and absorbing it, and weight-loss becomes almost impossible. Of course, weight-gain is also probable.

Magnesium, it turns out, can neutralize the effects of stress. It does this by supporting and feeding your adrenal glands, preventing your adrenal glands from becoming overworked, and helping you maintain a calm attitude.

Hopefully you're beginning to see that without adequate amounts of magnesium, you're bound to develop an irregular metabolism...and gain weight.

Will you be a person who finds that you can lose weight (or maintain your desired weight) just by practicing a magnesium-rich diet?

If you are ready, here's what to do:

Avoid refined grains like white flour, sugared cereals, muffins, bagels, or white rice, since these foods have nutrients like magnesium filtered out of them when they are processed.

Instead, fill your menu with foods high in magnesium, like fruits, vegetables (especially leafy green vegetables), beans, nuts, seeds, and fish.

How much magnesium should you include in your diet each day?

The Recommended Dietary Allowance (RDA) for magnesium is between 400 to 420 mg per day for adult males, and 310 to 320 mg per day for adult females. (The RDA for pregnant women is 350 mg to 360 mg per day.) But many experts believe you may need much more --- especially because of the Electric and Magnetic Fields (EMFs) you're subjected to daily.

EMFs have been shown to cause damage to human metabolic systems, and luckily magnesium can mitigate some of that damage.

So to have an adequate amount of magnesium, Dr. Mercola recommends that you include at least 1 to 2 grams (1,000 to 2,000 mg) of elemental magnesium per day.

Below is a guide which shows how much magnesium you can expect from a few organically-grown or naturally-sourced foods.

Magnesium amounts in organically-grown or naturally -sourced foods:

- Cooked spinach, 1 cup: 157 mg of magnesium
- Pumpkin Seeds, 1/4 cup (1 oz): 150 mg of magnesium
- Cooked Black Beans, 1 cup: 120 mg of magnesium
- Cooked Brown Rice, 1 cup: 84 mg of magnesium
- Cashew Nuts, 1/4 cup (1.3 oz): 82 mg of magnesium
- Baked Salmon, 3 oz: 19 mg of magnesium

I hope you're noticing the small amount of magnesium contained in each of the portions above.

Realistically then, to get adequate amounts you probably need to also take magnesium in a supplemental form. Labeling on magnesium capsules lets you know exactly how much magnesium is contained in each dose, and you can make sure you're getting as much as you need.

Today's Goal:

Determine which is the easiest way for you to take in at least the required daily quantity of magnesium: food form or supplement form. For real protection, and to realize your weight-loss goals, you might need a combination of the two.

You'll find many supplements on the market --- and can check out *www.kriswilliamswellness.com* for recommended magnesium brands.

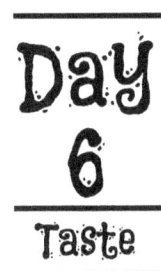

Day 6
Taste

MAGNESIUM POWDER WATER
(Serves 1)

Ingredients:

12 ounces filtered or spring water *(room temperature or slightly chilled)*
1 teaspoon powdered magnesium citrate
1 fresh lemon or lime wedge

Directions:

- Pour 12 ounces of filtered or spring water into a tall glass.
- Stir in 1 teaspoon of powdered magnesium.
- Squirt in juice from a lemon or lime ---
  (OR: add the magnesium to your apple cider vinegar/Manuka honey water.)
- Drink once or twice a day.
  (Your brain and muscles will thank you.)
- Enjoy!

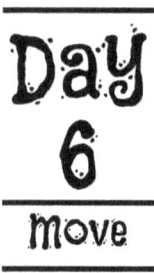

ISOMETRICS WHILE SITTING

Suck in your stomach.
Hold it for 5 seconds, then release.
Gradually increase to 10 seconds, then release.
Do this 10 times.

Tighten your buttocks.
Hold for 5 seconds, then release.
Gradually increase to 10 seconds, then release.
Do this 10 times.

Feel the energy run through your whole body.
Enjoy!

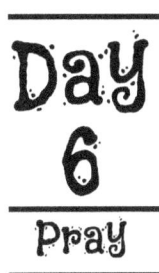

YOU KNOW ALL MY SECRETS

Hello God,

Help me to admit to you the things I do in secret:

I binge on cakes, cookies, donuts, chips, ice cream --- until I'm sick.

I wash down popcorn, pizza, burgers, tacos, and fries with sodas as if I have no self-control.

I think no one sees me.

But you do.

You say you are a God not only far away, but also nearby.

You say I can't hide from you in secret places,

Because you always see me...

Because you fill heaven and earth.

What I do in secret, let me admit to you.

Let me name these things --- so that I can begin to be healed.

And then give me the willingness to try this new way of controlling what I have up until now called "uncontrollable urges."

Show me easy ways to make sure I'm getting enough magnesium in my diet.

Jeremiah 23:23-24

"Am I only a God nearby,"
declares the Lord,
"and not a God far away?
Can anyone hide in secret places
so that I cannot see him[her]?"
declares the Lord.
"Do not I fill heaven and earth?"
declares the Lord.

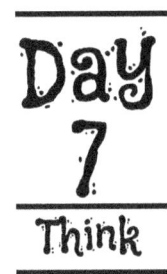

THE SECRET GARDEN

Good morning! Glad you're here today. I hope you've had a tall glass of refreshing water already --- perhaps with an invigorating portion of apple cider vinegar, a rounded teaspoon of powdered magnesium, and (if you need it) a small teaspoon of raw, unfiltered honey?

Good.

Then come on out back --- into the garden.

I've got some particular trees I'd like to show you.

I see the glint in your eye when you notice that I have quite a few fruit trees.

You're confused about why I grow them, especially after what I told you on your second day with me.

You wonder why I grow them because you think I don't eat much fruit.

You heard me say that fructose is a dangerous thief, and fruit is full of fructose.

Which is true.

Fruit is full of fructose.

So forgive me for the dilemma in which I might have left you.

May I repeat what I hope you heard on the second day?

It is the REFINED fructose, ADDED fructose, and MANUFACTURED FRUCTOSE SYRUPS like high fructose corn syrup (HFCS)--- as well as an OVERABUNDANCE of natural fructose --- that are the culprits which steal your health away.

ADDED sugars cause your skin to break out, your blood sugar to spike, your moods to swing, your joints to hurt, your heart to palpitate, your urinary tract to become infected, and your whole body to become inflamed. Large portions of fructose cause you to become ill. ADDED sugars of all kinds cause you to gain weight.

On the other hand, WHOLE fruits, in moderation, can be very healthy for you.

Eating a WHOLE fruit means that you are not just consuming the juice, but you're ingesting every part of the pod, berry, or drupe: the flesh, the fiber, and sometimes even the skin. The parts you might discard at times would be the hard rinds or the seeds.

Eating a WHOLE fruit supplies you with tiny "magic" compounds --- or micro-nutrients --- that can significantly affect your health for the better. When you find a place for whole fruits in your diet, you become ill less frequently, and it's easier to lose weight, maintain your desired weight, and call up energy that your body needs for mental and physical activity.

Here's a strange secret: your body is continually falling apart.

It's true.

Your body is continuously breaking down through a process known as oxidation.

Whenever you breathe, eat, or move, your body requires energy. In the process of using up energy, cells break down, and waste is produced.

Breakdowns in your body speed up when you eat the wrong things --- like poisonous arsenic and cyanide --- or when you eat what you might think of as innocent things --- like added sugars.

Arsenic and cyanide have the ability to break your body down quickly --- before they kill you.

Sugar works more slowly --- inflaming your joints and causing disease and obesity --- before leading to death.

What can you do to prevent the breakdown?

What can you do to stop your body from rusting, your joints from becoming inflamed, and the fat from being produced?

You can make sure you get a good supply of *anti*oxidants from the foods you eat.

Why?

Antioxidants help to keep your body from oxidizing --- or breaking down --- too quickly.

If your body is breaking down, you won't be able to lose weight and maintain your health.

Antioxidants contain compounds that have anti-inflammatory effects. When your body is inflamed, it won't regulate your hormones, digest your food, or efficiently get rid of your waste.

Antioxidants also work to keep all the machinery in your body running smoothly. Without antioxidants, your body doesn't get the signals it needs to properly digest and assimilate the foods you eat.

Without antioxidants, you don't have the energy to lose weight.

Remember this one forgotten secret to losing weight: *You need to eat to lose.*

And you need to make sure you eat the right things to lose the right amount of weight, and keep it off.

What constitute the "right" things?

Foods containing antioxidants.

And one terrific source of antioxidants is fruit.

So if you need antioxidants from food, more is better. Right?

Wrong. Here is where you need to think like Goldilocks. Just like Goldilocks wanted to find the right-size chair, the right-temperature porridge, and the perfectly-comfortable bed, you want to consume the amount of fruit that is "just right."

Two reasons why you don't want to overdose on fruit:
1. While your body is breaking down and producing free radicals (otherwise known as *oxidants* --- a small amount

of which your body does need to do its work), it is also manufacturing *anti*oxidants on its own to counteract the damaging effects of the oxidants! So your body already is providing some of the antioxidants you need to keep yourself healthy. In most cases, though, oxidants (or the bad-guy free-radicals) far outnumber the naturally occurring antioxidants (or the good-guy cleaner-uppers). Nevertheless, in today's world, your body could never produce enough antioxidants required to fight oxidation and inflammation.

2. The second reason you don't want to overdose on fruit is that fruit is high in fructose. (This is a great time to review Day 2!)

But fruit will help you to lose weight!

Fruits in general help you lose weight because of the generous amount of Vitamin-C they contain. Vitamin-C specifically works to help eliminate the dangerous fat cells that build up around your belly. When you don't have enough Vitamin-C, you're sabotaging your efforts to lose weight, even if you're exercising.

A study published in the *Nutrition & Metabolism (London) Journal* in 2006 revealed that people who exercised with low concentrations of Vitamin-C in their blood burned 25 percent less fat than other participants in the study who had adequate amounts in their blood. (Vitamin-C is crucial for manufacturing carnitine, a nifty little compound that helps burn fat so you can use it for energy.)

Another reason Vitamin-C is a valuable nutrient for weight-loss is that it hinders stress hormones from initiating fat storage around your belly area. Remember that when you are stressed, you release cortisol. Cortisol increases the production of insulin, and more insulin in your blood means more fat in your tissues. (Just a little more review from Day 2....!)

How much Vitamin-C do you really need each day?

The RDA is 90 mg for men and 75 mg for women. But many health practitioners recommend much more --- anywhere from four to eight to even 20 times as much.

Dr. Weil says that 120 to 200 mg seems to be the optimal amount for maintaining health and reversing chronic conditions. But if you live with a smoker, or in a smoggy town, or are otherwise highly stressed, he recommends taking up to 1,200 mg a day.

(Don't go overboard, though, with the amount of Vitamin-C you consume. More than 2,000 mg a day could cause diarrhea, abdominal cramps and nausea, according to the Office of Dietary Supplements.)

To get an idea about how much Vitamin-C is in whole fruits, see the following list:

- Strawberries, 1 cup: 85 mg
- Pineapple, 1 cup: 79 mg
- Kiwi, 1: 64 mg
- Bell Pepper (red, 1 cup chopped): 190 mg
- Bell Pepper (green, 1 cup chopped): 120 mg
- Bell Pepper (yellow, 1 cup chopped): 183 mg
- Bell Pepper (orange, 1 cup chopped): 128 mg
- Orange, 1 cup of sections: 83 mg

The key: Eat the whole fruit.

If you're anything like me, you're a beast when your hunger is out of control. You get cranky, irritable, impatient, and rude. You don't like people very much at those times, and you probably end up not liking yourself very much either. So you reach for the nearest, most convenient thing to satisfy your hunger...and stress or depression may make you keep on eating.

How do you get control of your hunger? How do you free yourself from becoming a slave to your hunger pangs? How do you make sure you're on the right road to losing weight?

You can control hunger pangs and stay on the road to losing weight by including a variety of fruits in your diet as you travel.

What fruits are best for hunger-control and weight-loss?

- **Citrus fruits** (in particular) help control hunger pangs because they neutralize the acid in your system. Less acid means less bloating, less inflammaton, and higher energy levels. When energy levels are high, you don't go looking for more to eat to "pick you up."

- **Citrus fruits** (in particular) help you lose weight because they contain high amounts of Vitamin-C.

- **Lemons, limes, grapefruits, and oranges** are citrus fruits that aid in the elimination of toxins from your organs --- particularly your liver --- one of your major detox organs. When your liver is clean and functioning efficiently, you are better able to assimilate the foods you take in, and you're better able to eliminate their waste once the foods are digested.

  Lemons, limes, grapefruits, and oranges also promote good bowel movement --- which is the last step in waste removal from your body.

  Proper digestion and elimination of toxins from your organs, plus regular removal of waste from your intestines, lead to healthy weight-loss.

Other fruits that aid in weight-loss:

- **Fresh raspberries, blackberries, cranberries, strawberries, and blueberries** are very helpful in weight-loss for three reasons: they're low in calories, high in water, and high in fiber. Such foods are known as low-energy-dense foods. *Raspberries could be a particularly good choice when you're trying to lose weight because of substances they contain called ketones. Ketones boost metabolism, and in studies where rats ate raspberry ketones, the ketones prevented the rats' total body fat from increasing. Ketones were especially effective in burning the dangerous and deep-seated internal belly fat of those animals. (I don't want to get your hopes up too high on this weight-loss trick, though, because research is still ongoing for the same ketone-response in humans...)*

Berries are considered very effective fruits in aiding weight-loss because they can help to control the insulin response in your body. A cup of strawberries before a meal, for instance, could help reduce your blood sugar and insulin levels after meals. Researchers surmise that it's the antioxidants present in strawberries which slow down digestive enzymes. Slowing down digestion means that food particles stay longer in your blood, keeping your insulin levels even, and helping to keep you satiated so that you don't overeat.

- **Melons**
  Fruits such as watermelon, cantaloupe, musk melon, and honeydew melon all contain a high amount of water --- with a lesser amount of carbohydrates (or sugars).

  Eating fruits with lots of water will always improve your digestion, making it easier to eliminate waste from your body.

  What about watermelon? Isn't watermelon high in sugar? Yes, but...

  Yes, it's true that with one cup of chopped watermelon you'll be ingesting 5.1 grams of fructose, so it is important to factor this number into your 15-grams-a-day limit for fructose.

  But one cup contains only 46 calories. And also in that one cup of chopped watermelon, there is a small amount of protein, a measurable amount of fiber, several antioxidants, and one added weight-loss benefit: watermelon contains an amino acid (one of the building blocks of protein) called L-citrulline.

  L-citrulline is converted in your body to another amino acid called L-arginine which --- because it activates nitric oxide --- increases blood circulation to all of your organs and skin. When your blood is circulating well, your immune and digestive systems function better. When your immune and digestive systems function better, you amp up your ability to fight infection and digest food. With those systems working well, you're able to lose weight more easily.

L-arginine is also being shown to aid in weight-loss by burning excess fat (as well as improving muscle mass!)

From various animal studies, scientists suggest that L-arginine reduces fat mass by increasing insulin activity. How? By way of influencing hormones that are involved in fat metabolism.

One peculiar rule for melons: *Eat them alone or leave them alone.* You digest melons more easily when eaten separately from other fruits and foods.

- **Peppers:**
Would you have guessed that peppers are fruits? (They are.) Would you have guessed that mild peppers burn calories, just like hot peppers do? (They do.) Sweet red and green peppers (along with hot chilis) contain 2 metabolism-boosting ingredients:
1. *Vitamin-C.* One cup of chopped bell peppers provides you with two times the USDA's recommended allowance.
2. *Dihydrocapsiate.* This compound works like capsaicin to speed up metabolism and cause the body to burn fat instead of other energy stores. (You're going to find out more about capsaicin on Day 12.)

Want to lose weight by doing nothing more than eating?

Consume 2 portions of fruit each day.

"One portion" consists of either 1 piece of whole fruit (such as an apple) or one cup of chopped fruit (such as watermelon or berries). Remember that you're going to find higher levels of polyphenols (antioxidants) in the outer layers of the plants than you will in the inner parts. So eat the whole fruit.

Peppers, by the way, are one food you can have as many servings of as you want!

When's the best time to eat fruit?

Mornings are a perfect time to incorporate portions of fruit into your diet. The reason why is that this is the time of day when your body is most efficient at eliminating its waste products, and fruits encourage elimination. A morning fruit shake will provide some of the liquid you need in your day. Plus, it may just put a smile on your face, and being happy allows your body to do its best work.

Remember: don't get carried away.

Consider the positives of fruit:

- Fruit contains high amounts of water.
- Fruit contains good fiber.
- Fruit contains antioxidants.
- Many fruits contain substances that enhance health and even further enhance weight-loss.
- Fruit tastes good to eat!

Consider the negative of fruit:

- Many fruits contain high amounts of fructose. Consume wisely.

By the way, I also hope you're continuing to read the labels of the foods and drinks before you buy. If so, are you noticing something surprising? Are you noticing that bottled juice usually contains added sugar and/or high-fructose corn syrup (HFCS)?

If you've ever ordered a fruit smoothie at a commercial shop, did you notice how the vendor filled up your cup with sugar-laden canned fruits or juice without any fiber, instead of using fresh, whole fruit and no additional sugars...?

Weight-Loss Secret #7:

Replace your canned soda and commercial fruit juice smoothies with one or two pieces/servings of whole fruit.

During our time together, I'm suggesting that your total grams of fructose from fruit should be below 15 grams per day.

You can plan your daily intake using the following chart showing how many **grams of fructose** are contained in the amount of fruit listed:

- Limes: 1 medium = 0
- Lemons: 1 medium = 0.6
- Cranberries: 1 cup = 0.63
- Passion fruit: 1 medium = 0.9
- Guava: 1 medium = 1.1
- Prune : 1 medium = 1.2
- Apricot : 1 medium = 1.3
- Date (Deglet Noor style): 1 medium = 2.6
- Cantaloupe: 1/8 medium melon = 2.8
- Raspberries: 1 cup = 3.0
- Clementine: 1 medium = 3.4
- Kiwifruit: 1 medium = 3.4
- Blackberries: 1 cup = 3.5
- Star fruit: 1 medium = 3.6
- Strawberries: 1 cup (sliced) = 4
- Cherries, sweet: 10 = 3.8
- Cherries, sour: 1 cup = 4.0
- Pineapple: 1 cup (chunks) = 4.0
- Grapefruit (pink or red): ½ medium = 4.3
- Apple (Granny Smith): 1 medium = 5.0
- Watermelon: 1 cup (diced) = 5.1
- Nectarine: 1 medium = 5.4
- Peach: 1 medium = 5.9
- Orange (Navel): 1 medium = 6.1
- Papaya: ½ medium = 6.3
- Honeydew: 1/8 medium = 6.7

- Banana: 1 medium = 7.1
- Blueberries: 1 cup = 7.4
- Fig: 1 medium = 8
- Apple (composite): 1 medium = 9.5
- Grapes: 1 cup = 12.4
- Mango: 1/2 medium = 16.2

Fructose in dried fruit is much more concentrated.

For instance:

- Dried figs: 1/2 cup = 17 grams
- Dried cranberries: 1/2 cup = 22 grams
- Raisins: 1/2 cup = 24 grams

Looking at these super-sized amounts of fructose should make you want to avoid dried fruits during your 21-day journey --- especially because they are devoid of any life-giving water --- and especially now while you're trying to get your insulin, your cravings, and your weight under control.

How much fruit are you consuming?

Today's Goal:

Make a pact with yourself to eat two servings of whole fruit.

If you want a fruit juice or fruit smoothie, cut up a whole piece of fruit (or use whole berries) and liquify it (or them) in a blender. (No added sugar, please.) By ingesting the entire fruit, you'll be able to enjoy all of its benefits.

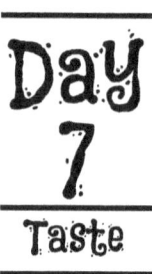

BLUEBERRY BLEND SMOOTHIE
(Serves 2)

Ingredients:

1 cup frozen blueberries *(pesticide-free)*
6 medium frozen strawberries *(pesticide-free)*
3-inch piece of peeled banana *(fresh or frozen)*
1/2 cup coconut water
1 cup purified or spring water
1 handful fresh basil, washed

Directions:

- Put all of the above ingredients into a blender, blend on medium-to-high speed for 15 seconds.

Then:

- Divide the resulting smoothie into 2 glasses if you will be drinking one glass immediately and sharing the other;
  (otherwise, pour your 2nd divided amount into a glass jar, seal it with a lid, and keep it for tomorrow.)
- Remember to chew each mouthful of your smoothie.
- For now, use this as the first "food" of the day. *(If you can wait until 10 or 11 o'clock in the morning to drink this, all the better.)*
- Enjoy!

Day 7
move

CHEW

Chew your juice.
Take one sip…
Swirl the liquid around your mouth…
Taste what you're swirling…
Chew.

Go ahead and laugh!
But then remember:
Digestion begins in the mouth.
Enjoy each mouthful!

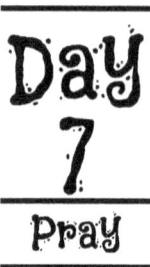

Day 7
Pray

WHY DO I INSIST ON CONSUMING WHAT ISN'T GOOD FOR MY BODY?

Hello God,

In the 55th chapter of Isaiah, you ask me why I spend money on food that doesn't give me strength, and why I labor for what will not satisfy me.

And I'll tell you:

I do it because the foods that do me no good are so available, and they're so tempting. With them I get instant gratification. They're foods that are full of sweetness and softness and made ready-to-eat! I keep laboring to fill up my grocery bag or cart with them --- even though they don't satisfy me --- because I have to admit, I'm addicted to them.

But right now --- I don't want to be addicted.

How do I free myself from this addiction?

You said that every good gift is from you.

But you also know that I have a wayward bent, and am prone to misuse the good gifts you give.

So let me begin to change the pattern by giving something back to you: my ear.

You ask me to listen to you.

So I will listen as you tell me what my body and soul need.

You promise that I will delight in the richest of fare.

WHY DO I INSIST ON CONSUMING WHAT ISN'T GOOD FOR MY BODY?

Really?
I am listening now.
Give me a taste for fresh fruits that come from the trees of life.
But fill me up not just with food, but also with your words ---
so that my soul --- as well as my body --- will live.

Isaiah 55:2-3

Why spend money on what is not bread,
and your labor on what does not satisfy?
Listen, listen to me, and eat what is good,
and you will delight in the richest of fare.
Give ear and come to me;
listen, that you may live.

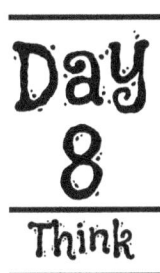

SECRET WEAPON #8 IN THE BATTLE OF THE BULGE:
FREE FOODS

You probably figured that, eventually, I'd show you the vegetable garden.

And perhaps you've been dreading what you thought I was going to say about the edibles that grow there.

That they're necessary.

That they're important.

That you've gotta eat them…

to lose weight and all. To be healthy.

Maybe you haven't always been keen on vegetables.

When you were growing up, someone stood over you wagging a finger declaring that you had to eat all your vegetables before you could have dessert.

Which made eating them like some sort of punishment.

What a shame.

Because a vegetable can be a dessert…a dessert that you can eat as much of as you want. And still be healthy. And still lose weight.

The difference between a vegetable "dessert" and the kind of desserts you're used to is the difference between **"free"** food and **"expensive"** food.

Expensive foods are those things you eat in the present --- those things that put a smile on your face as you eat them --- but that end up costing you your health in the future. The price you have to pay for expensive foods is: bloating, headaches, mood swings, stiff joints, diabetes, heart disease, liver disease, Alzheimer's disease, cancer...and weight gain that leads to obesity.

One type of *expensive* food is the type that comes with added sugars: sodas, bottled fruit juices, commercial ice cream, commercially packaged yogurt, commercial cereals, canned foods, packaged dinners, crackers, cookies, cakes, pies, donuts, and coffee-shop razzle-dazzle drinks.

When you're trying to lose weight you always need **"free"** foods!

"Free" means any food that you can eat as much of as you want, any time you want.

But **"free"** does come with guidelines, and for a food to qualify as **"free,"** it must fit into the following guidelines:

- **"Free"** food has a respectable amount of fiber and a low amount of calories.
- **"Free"** food isn't going to hurt you.
- **"Free"** food is going to do you some good.
- **"Free"** food takes time to chew, and fills you up so that you have less time and less inclination to chow down on high-calorie, thieving, dangerous, high-risk, cancer-causing, fat-producing, "expensive" foods.

Which vegetables are "free" foods?

"Free" foods include these botanical fruits that you usually think of as vegetables:

- eggplant
- okra
- zucchini
- cucumbers
- bell peppers (green, red, yellow)

These stem vegetables:

- celery
- asparagus

- rhubarb
- fennel

These leafy vegetables:
- Brussel sprouts
- cabbage
- lettuce
- kale
- spinach
- Swiss chard

These bud vegetables:
- cauliflower
- artichoke
- broccoli

These two root vegetables:
- radish
- onions

This one pod vegetable:
- green beans

I hope I'm not bursting your bubble when I tell you that starchy pod vegetables like peas, and root vegetables like beets, turnips, and rutabagas are not "free." But they're not "expensive," either. Pod and root vegetables are generally good for you, but if you want to maintain your weight, you should eat them by portion-size (because of their sugar and starch content).

Two particular root vegetables --- carrots and potatoes --- are not "free," but they are *"cheap"*!

"What are *"cheap"* foods?" you ask.

I'll tell you.

"Cheap" foods are those foods that won't cost you your weight-loss goals if you eat a lot of them...*IF* you prepare them or eat them

the right way. (You can find out how to prepare and eat **"cheap"** vegetables at the end of your reading for today.)

Remember:

You can and should eat as many green vegetables a day as you'd like.

Eat them alone or with a bit of salt and pepper.

Fix them in a salad and add a little olive oil, balsamic vinaigrette, salt, and pepper. (No bottled salad dressings, please. I'll tell you why on Day 15.)

Eat them with a bit of organic almond butter or peanut butter (without added sugar).

Dip them into a little hummus.

Add variety to your meals and snacks by choosing different vegetables for your salads or for cooking each week. Doing this will keep your taste-buds curiously satisfied and your body a thankful vessel for all the healthy polyphenols you're feeding it. Besides, eating one-vegetable-only for weeks at a time might cause a build-up of one specific mineral in your system, and leave you lacking in others.

Here from my list of **"free"** vegetables are reasons why (besides the fact that they taste good!) you can and should add them to your healthy weight-loss diet at any time:

CUCUMBERS are a great weight-loss food because:

- Cucumbers are high in water. There's little science behind the rule that says every person should drink eight 8-ounce glasses of water daily. But there *is* a lot of science behind the guideline advising every person to remain hydrated all day long. Each person's requirement for the amount of water he or she needs is different, but every cell of your body, along with every cell of every other human being on our planet, is about 60% water. You are meant to be --- created to be --- filled up with life-giving water.
One of the reasons I've emphasized drinking a glass of water first thing in the morning and before each meal

SECRET WEAPON #8 IN THE BATTLE OF THE BULGE:

is that I want to make sure you're taking in *at least* four 8-ounce glasses of water daily. Drinking water when you wake up and before each time you eat is helping you form a habit.

You're programming your body to look forward to becoming hydrated at specific times.

Water is essential if you:

Don't want to be constipated.
Don't want to develop kidney stones.
Want your body to move without hurting.
Want your body to experience less fatigue.
Want your brain to function accurately.
Want your mood to stay in balance.
Want fewer or no headaches.
Want to prevent a hangover.
Want to lose weight.

Since cucumbers are 96% water, one medium cucumber could count for at least ½ cup of water in your day.

- Cucumbers are high in fiber. The soluble fiber in cucumbers liquefies into gelatin in your digestive system, and this substance slows down your digestion, which is a good thing. When absorption is slowed, your blood sugar doesn't spike and crash, and you end up feeling full longer. (We'll talk more about the importance of fiber --- for your health and for weight-loss --- on Day 14.)

- The mix of vitamins in cucumbers includes Vitamin-B1 (thiamine), Vitamin-B5 (pantothenic acid), and Vitamin-B7 (biotin). B vitamins have been shown to relieve anxiety and to guard a person against the damaging effects of stress, two predicaments you want to avoid when you're trying to lose weight.

- Cucumbers make a great base for vegetable juices. Some nutritionists suggest that certain people can build up too much oxalic acid (and as a result form kidney stones) or are in danger of having their thyroid gland grow excessive tissue (known as a goiter) if they consume large amounts

SECRET WEAPON #8 IN THE BATTLE OF THE BULGE:

of green vegetables or certain nuts and seeds. This is one reason given for rotating the plants you eat. My advice: try not to eat the same veggies day after day. Cucumbers are no cause for worry, though. You can consume them regularly, without cost.

CELERY is a great weight-loss food because:

- A single, large stalk of celery contains only 10 calories, and a cup of chopped raw celery adds up to a mere 16 calories.
- But celery is more than just a low-calorie food. It's high in Vitamin-K, Vitamin-A, Vitamin-B9 (folic acid), Vitamin-B6 (pyridoxine), Vitamin-C, and potassium. Celery contains certain antioxidants and polysaccharides that reduce stress (caused by your body's breaking down) that can lead to inflammation.
- Unlike some vegetables, celery retains most of its nutrients even if it's steamed.
- Celery is also a good source of fiber (but only if you're eating it or putting it into a smoothie --- not if you're juicing it. We'll talk more about the importance of fiber --- for your health and for weight-loss --- on Day 14.)

GREEN BEANS are a great weight-loss food because:

- Besides containing a reasonable amount of Vitamin-C and Vitamin-K, green beans have a high amount of iron. Your cardiovascular system needs iron for the formation of hemoglobin, the protein that carries oxygen through your bloodstream. You also need iron to help produce the energy your cells use to function properly and your metabolism requires to run efficiently. How much iron do you need daily? If you're a man, you only need 8 milligrams. If you're a woman, you need 18 milligrams. Eating one cup of string beans will provide you with 1 milligram of iron.
- Green beans are also high in fiber. The fiber in green beans can not only prevent weight-gain, but can also promote weight-loss. (More fiber-rich treasures for you to discover on Day 14.)

SECRET WEAPON #8 IN THE BATTLE OF THE BULGE:

ZUCCHINI is a great weight-loss food because:

- Besides fiber, zucchini is high in vitamins, minerals, antioxidants, and water, and low in calories. Yay! A free food!
- Did you know that because of zucchini's high water content (it's 95% water), when you eat it, you end up with more energy and fewer headaches?
- Zucchini's Vitamin-A keeps your eyes healthy so you can see what you're eating, its Vitamin-C is good for fighting asthma so you can breathe easily, and zucchini's calcium keeps your teeth fortified so you can continue to chew the foods that give you better health --- and help you lose weight.

CAULIFLOWER is a great weight-loss food because:

- "When you're looking for foods that are going to keep you fuller for longer, look for ones high in fiber, healthy fats, and protein, or with a high water content," says Barbara Rolls, Ph.D., professor of nutrition at Penn State University and author of *The Volumetrics Eating Plan (1999)*.
And one of the few foods that can be eaten in unlimited quantities is cauliflower, Dr. Rolls says. The reason why cauliflower may be especially helpful for weight-loss is that it comes packaged with Vitamin-C --- the nutrient that is key in how much fat you burn during physical activity. (But, as I mentioned earlier, don't go overboard with the amount of Vitamin-C you consume; more than 2,000 mg a day could cause diarrhea, abdominal cramps, and nausea, according to the Office of Dietary Supplements. One cup of raw, chopped cauliflower contains about 52 mg of Vitamin-C.)

I have space right here to repeat this often overlooked secret to weight management once more: When you are mentally and physically healthy, you lose weight --- and maintain your weight --- more easily.

Cruciferous vegetables contribute to making and keeping you healthy.

SECRET WEAPON #8 IN THE BATTLE OF THE BULGE:

Professionals recommend cruciferous vegetables for health because of their ability to deliver a variety of vitamins, minerals, proteins, carbohydrates, and fats that are needed to keep all seven of your body systems functioning in top condition. When your immune system, inflammatory system, cardiovascular system, hormonal system, detoxification system, digestive system, and/or antioxidant system function poorly, the possibility of your cells becoming cancerous dramatically increases. Cruciferous vegetables are able to aid in the proper functioning of all seven of these systems.

Cruciferous vegetables also stand out because they're full of phytonutrients (another name for plant nutrients that include carotenoids and flavonoids). Phytonutrients perform subtle but pivotal functions in the creation of your strength and energy.

My list of *cruciferous* vegetables that will work to keep you healthy in every way possible:

- Broccoli
- Cabbage
- Kale
- Collard Greens
- Brussels Sprouts
- Cauliflower
- Bok Choy
- Mustard Greens
- Turnip
- Watercress
- Rutabaga
- Horseradish
- Daikon Radish/Radish
- Wasabi

SECRET WEAPON #8 IN THE BATTLE OF THE BULGE:

Two *cruciferous* vegetables that are "free" foods, and that will specifically help with weight-loss:

BROCCOLI

Besides protecting you against prostate, breast, lung, and skin cancers, *this bud vegetable can also help you achieve what you're after: weight-loss.*

Broccoli does this in two ways:

1. *Through Vitamin-C.*
   Vitamin-C is able to help you when you're stressed by lowering your cortisol levels. Cortisol is a hormone that increases in your system when you're stressed, causing you to store fat. With reduced cortisol levels, less fat will be stored --- specifically less fat around your belly area. Plus, a little bit of broccoli goes a long way. Eating only a small amount of broccoli (one cup, chopped) can give you the Vitamin-C you need for the day.

2. *Through a phytonutrient called sulforaphane.*
   Sulforaphane in broccoli has been shown to increase testosterone levels and attack fat storage (besides attacking cancer cells). Testosterone is one of those hormones that help build muscle, and the more muscle mass you have, the more calories you burn while you're resting!

   (Beware that sometimes broccoli can give people with sensitive stomachs bouts of gas. The more your system adjusts to eating vegetables, however, the more it will be able to digest well the vegetables you eat. Until then, check out *www.kriswilliamswellness.com* for brands of gentle digestive enzymes.)

KALE

Kale works to keep you healthy while aiding in weight-loss in six ways:

1. *Through a high content of Vitamin-C.*
   Kale has more Vitamin-C than oranges. One medium orange contains 113% of the RDA for Vitamin-C, while

one cup of chopped kale contains 134%. And remember, for weight-loss, you're looking to reduce your stress in any way possible. Vitamin-C fights stress.

2. *Through Vitamin-A.*
Low intakes of vitamin-A can result in poor vision, dry skin, impaired reproduction, impaired growth, decreased energy, and increased susceptibility to infection. For weight-loss, you're looking to keep your body healthy and energetic, and Vitamin-A is a natural, constant infection-fighter. One cup of chopped kale will provide you with 206 percent of your daily need for Vitamin-A.

3. *Through phytonutrients called isothiocyanates.*
Isothiocyanates (made from glucosinolates) increase your body's detoxifying power. Poisons wandering around in your body cause the death of cells --- leading to poor energy production, and the malfunction of your liver, kidneys, and brain. Kale is able to clean out pesticides and other environmental poisons that come with processed foods and the drugs you might be taking. (Glucosinolates trigger your liver to produce detoxifying enzymes that block damage from free-radical poisons.)

4. *Through its content of thylakoids.*
Thylakoids help fight sugar cravings by slowing the digestive process and promoting proper communication among your hormones, both of which keep your blood sugar in check and tell your brain you're full.

5. *Through the power of fiber…which also helps you feel full.*
For the last seven days, you've been paying attention to what thirst feels like. And you've also been paying attention to what hunger feels like.
Now it's time to pay attention to what it feels like to be "full." Kale can fill you up in a satisfying way.

6. *Through a high calcium content.*
Kale has a higher percentage of usable calcium than spinach. Spinach is actually considered by many to be a

poor source of calcium because its bioavailability is poor. The oxalic acid in spinach prevents you from absorbing more than about 10% --- or about 24.5mg --- of the 245mg of calcium from one cup of cooked spinach. So even though a serving of kale (1 cup, cooked) contains just 197mg of calcium, about 50% of it is bioavailable --- which means that you'd end up with about 96mg of calcium that your body could actually use.

(By the way, your body is able to absorb only 30-35% of all the available calcium in cow's milk and dairy products. This means that if there are 300 mg of calcium present in a 1-cup serving of milk, you'll be able to absorb only 90 to 105mg. The rest leaves your body mainly in your urine and feces.)

Calcium has a starring role in determining bone density, muscle contraction, nerve function, blood pressure stability, and healing. If you're ill or hurt, you don't want to think about your weight goals. I know. It's easy to use being sick or injured as an excuse. I've done it.

Instead, make kale a regular addition to your diet.

Kale Caution:

Kale is often on the Environmental Working Group's (EWG) dirty dozen list of vegetables, which means it's most likely to have lots of pesticide residue if grown conventionally. So I recommend choosing organic kale, if at all possible.

Two *leafy green vegetables* that are "free" foods, and that will specifically help with weight-loss:

SPINACH

- Spinach helps with weight-loss because, surprisingly, it has protein.
- Whether you steam one cup of it or throw one cup of it into your blender to add to a smoothie, you'll be getting as much protein as a medium hard-boiled egg. Protein bolsters muscle growth, and if you're exercising with weights, protein aids muscle recovery as well.

SECRET WEAPON #8 IN THE BATTLE OF THE BULGE:

What's the advantage to weight-loss when you exercise to build muscle? This is a repeat from above, but it's good to be reminded: the more muscle mass you have, the more calories you burn while you're resting.

- Besides protein, this leafy green powerhouse is home to Vitamin-K, Vitamin-A, manganese, Vitamin-B9 (folate), magnesium, iron, copper, Vitamin-B2 (riboflavin), Vitamin-B6 (pyridoxine), Vitamin-E, calcium, Vitamin-C, potassium, fiber, Vitamin-B1 (thiamine), phosphorus, zinc, choline, omega-3 fats, Vitamin-B3 (niacin), selenium, and Vitamin-B5 (pantothenic acid). You see what I mean about the good you can do to yourself when you eat a vegetable?

- The added kicker for weight-loss: spinach contains *thylakoids*, those compounds which have been shown to help reduce sugar cravings. I know you've had to fight sugar cravings whenever you've tried to lose extra pounds in the past. Did you ever consider that you were victim to those sugar cravings in the first place because you weren't eating the right nutrients? Who would have thought that eating more would curb your enthusiasm for sugar?
  In a few minutes, I'm going to give you a simple recipe that includes spinach --- to put you on a new path which will help you fight cravings naturally.

ROMAINE LETTUCE

- Romaine lettuce helps with weight-loss because it's extremely low in calories and high in water.

- Romaine lettuce is also packed with hunger-fighting, health-giving compounds like Vitamin-C, beta-carotene, Vitamin-K, Vitamin-B9 (folate), and manganese. It is also one of the best dietary sources of chromium. What foresight God demonstrated when He tucked Vitamin-C into romaine lettuce. We've already talked about Vitamin-C's capacity to fight stress, but we haven't spoken about Vitamin-C's second super-power: its ability to enhance the absorption of chromium.
  Chromium is significant in weight-loss because it can help

increase your lean-body mass, or maintain a lean-body mass that you already have (when you combine chromium with exercise). Scientists think that chromium helps to make you leaner because of its capacity to keep you sensitive to insulin. When your body continues to respond to insulin, less sugar is stored as fat --- especially fat around your midsection.

- *(Alert: Because romaine lettuce has been listed as one of the foods having a pretty high risk of E. coli contamination, choosing an organic brand and washing it thoroughly before eating are recommended.)*

Two vegetables high(er) in sugar and/or starch than other vegetables listed here, but still available to eat "cheaply:"

CARROTS

- Carrots are great for weight-loss because of their fiber content. Fiber helps to keep you feeling fuller longer and prevents you from overeating at future meals.
Pectin is the main digestible fiber in carrots, beneficial because it slows down the digestion of a carrot's sugar and starch.
Other digestible fibers in carrots work in your digestive tract to hinder cholesterol from being absorbed into your blood --- which means that carrots help lower your blood cholesterol.
Non-digestible fiber helps to prevent constipation --- and we'll talk more about why it's important to have regular bowel movements on Day 14.

- Besides fiber, carrots come packed with beta-carotene, Vitamin-K, potassium, and antioxidants, and they have a good portion of water.

- Eat carrots raw or cooked, but drink no more than one cup of carrot *juice* per day. One cup can contain up to 14 grams of sugar, and juicing extracts the fiber, so there's nothing left to moderate the speed in which the carrot's sugar is absorbed into your blood. (Still, raw or cooked carrots are a cheap food you can eat often. Just make sure you chew each bite at least...15 times!)

POTATOES: Boil or roast them and eat them only after they've been cooled (and reheated, if you prefer).

- Potato starch is what makes potatoes weight-loss-friendly. The weight-loss quality is activated only if you eat the potatoes after they've been cooked and then cooled. You can reheat them later.
  Here's what happens after potatoes have cooled:
  Their digestible starches turn into "resistant starches" --- through a chemical process that actually enables them to resist digestion in your gut. While the potatoes are "resisting," they're promoting the oxidation (or breakdown) of fat around your middle.

- Important heads-up: don't fry potatoes in vegetable oils! (You'll find out how these oils are sabotaging your health and weight-loss goals on Day 17.)

Today's Goal:

Eat at least 5 servings of vegetables.

Can you do it?

One serving is about the size of your fist, if you're a woman, and the size of two fists, if you're a man. (How interesting it is that the One who created you allows you to measure with your own hand the amount that could be just right for you!)

If you feel you need another kind of measurement, one serving is about one cup of chopped vegetable.

Ways to include 5 vegetables in your diet in one day:

- Put 2 servings in a smoothie...
- Eat a salad with 3 servings for lunch...
- Have a small salad and a vegetable for dinner...

Day 8
Taste

SWISS BLISS GREEN DRINK
(Serves 2)

Ingredients:

- 1 large English cucumber *(peeled if you cannot use organic)*
- 1 large leaf Swiss chard
- 2 large stalks celery
- 2 handfuls spinach
- 2 medium oranges *(peeled)*
- ½ lemon *(peeled)*
- 6 English walnut halves

Directions:

- Clean and/or chop: *cucumber, Swiss chard, celery, oranges, & lemon.*
- Put *cucumber, Swiss chard, celery, oranges, & lemon* through a juicer, then:
- Pour juice into a blender and add *spinach & walnuts.*
  (If your blender is a mighty one, put peeled oranges & lemon in the blender with the spinach & walnuts.)
- Blend everything together on medium-high speed for 25-30 seconds.
- Pour into 2 glasses or glass jars.
  (Refrigerate in a sealed jar for no more than 48 hours.)
- Remember to "chew" each sip.
- Enjoy!

(Use the above recipe if you have not yet accustomed yourself to drinking vegetable smoothies. Otherwise, please check www.kriswilliamswellness.com for how to prepare the smoothie recipe.)

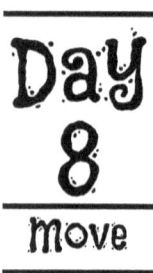

ISOMETRICS WHILE SITTING: LEGS

Move forward in your chair so that your feet are flat on the floor.

Extend your right leg in front of you (which you should be able to do under a desk).

Point your toe and hold for 5 seconds.

Flex your foot and hold for 5 seconds.

Return your right foot back flat on the floor.

Extend your left leg in front of you.

Point your toe and hold for 5 seconds.

Flex your foot and hold for 5 seconds.

Return your left foot back flat on the floor.

Gradually lift both legs, so you're extending them straight from your hips --- parallel with the floor. Hold for 5 seconds.

You'll notice that your stomach muscles are put to use, and you'll be tightening them automatically.

Repeat each leg and double lifts 5 times.

Feel the energy run through your whole body.

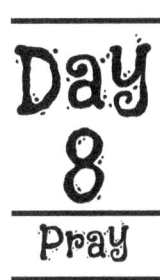

MY MIND IS A POWERFUL TOOL

Hello God,

I understand that achieving a healthy weight means that I might have to eat more vegetables...but so often I say to myself: *I don't wanna...*

Help me to understand that achieving a healthy weight isn't just about what I feed my body. It's also about what I feed my mind...It's also about the words I say to myself.

Spur me to change the negative phrases that run through my mind regularly.

Help me to change this sentence:

There's so much information to sift through in order to figure out what I should and shouldn't eat that I am overwhelmed.

To this:

Learning one new fact a day about health can make living my life more interesting, happier, and healthier.

Help me to change this sentence:

Vegetables are boring. They don't taste good to me.

To this:

I can try one new vegetable a week, prepare it in different ways, and see if I can come to like it.

Help me to change this sentence:

I don't have the time to shop for vegetables every day! Plus, they cost a lot of money, and they just go to waste.

To this:

Shopping for fresh vegetables means I spend less time and less money at the doctor's office.

Or this:

Shopping for fresh vegetables means I spend less money on packaged, processed foods, and end up saving money as I plan my meals.

Help me to change this sentence:

Cleaning or chopping fresh vegetables takes too much time.

To this:

Cleaning or chopping fresh vegetables takes less and less time each time I do it.

Help me to change this sentence:

I'm too tired to follow a plan!

To this:

I know that if I eat health-giving vegetables, I'll enjoy more time to plan, more money to use, and more energy to do the work you called me to do here on this earth.

Philippians 4:8
Finally, brothers and sisters,
whatever is true, whatever is noble, whatever is right,
whatever is pure, whatever is lovely,
whatever is admirable —
if anything is excellent or praiseworthy —
think about such things.

Romans 12:2
Do not be conformed to this world,
but be transformed by the renewal of your mind,
that by testing you may discern what is the will of God,
what is good and acceptable and perfect.

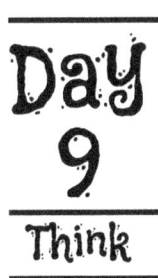

SMALL CHANGE, MIGHTY DIFFERENCE

I'm so glad you're back again today because I wanted to make sure you got the chance to investigate another corner of the garden that most people ordinarily ignore: the herb garden. It's a patch of ground you really ought to become familiar with if you're serious about becoming lean and free. I'm anxious for you to meet some particular herbs that grow here because each one is a miniature powerhouse which can make a mighty difference in your drinks, your foods, your body, and your life.

An enriched life is mostly about the little things:

Small acts of kindness.

Encouraging words like "You're a great example for me."

Short, hard words like "I was wrong" and "I'm sorry."

Appreciative words like "Thank you for serving me."

A few extra minutes spent listening.

A few extra minutes spent helping.

And the seasonings you add to your food and drinks.

Each of these minuscule things adds enrichment to the lives of others around you, and to your own life.

Ginger was an herb I spent little time with as a child. It lived at the back of our spice cabinet and was brought out only once during the year: at holiday time when it perked up recipes for cookies and breads.

Little did I know then about the healthful benefits available in fresh or powdered ginger. And only later did I find out about ginger's ability to help you lose weight.

The unique fragrance and sweet-tart flavor of ginger come from its natural oils, the most important of which is gingerol. And gingerol is the component responsible for many of ginger's medicinal qualities, which include improving the function of your brain, protecting yourself against Alzheimer's disease, and helping you lose weight.

(It turns out that ginger is more than just a little thing...!)

1. The first difference you'll notice after you add ginger to your vegetable juices or smoothies is that it draws out the full flavors of the ingredients while at the same time awakening your taste buds to their sweetness.

2. The second difference --- which you might not notice right away --- is that ginger can cure nausea and indigestion. It does this by helping your digestive tract assimilate all the nutrients your drink contains --- all the nutrients you're taking in --- so that you can be healthy, maintain your weight, or lose the extra pounds that have stubbornly stuck by your side for all these months or years.

But what I really wanted to share with you is how small amounts of this herb can help you lose weight in a big way.

3. Ginger promotes a thermogenic effect. In other words, it creates heat.

    The foods or particles from your drinks that you consume don't just sit there in your stomach. They naturally trigger a breakdown process in your body which requires energy. Right away your body starts expending energy to digest those food and drink particles, absorb them, and then distribute all useable nutrients to needy cells throughout your body. Expending energy creates heat, and expending energy also burns up calories.

    (Did you know your body utilizes more energy --- or calories --- to process proteins, than it does to digest and assimilate carbohydrates or fats? Find out more on Days 19 and 20.)

As it turns out, ginger can increase the production of heat in your body. It does this by gently speeding up your metabolism. A heated metabolism works faster and to work faster you need more energy. You've got to burn calories to provide more energy and more calories burned mean more pounds lost!

4. Ginger can help stop your bad-food cravings --- by stabilizing your blood sugar.

    (You'll notice that I mention the importance of stabilizing your blood sugar a lot in this guide because I want you to make this your goal.)

    I set the following words down for you with kind concern:

    Do all you can to stabilize your blood sugar. Only then can your mind, body, and emotions work together to lose weight, maintain your desired weight, or increase your energy.

    When you have frequent fluctuations in blood sugar, cravings increase for sugary drinks, desserts, snacks, and other highly processed foods that are addictive. The hormone that naturally lets you know you're satisfied after a meal (leptin) goes wacko, and you feel hungry soon after you've eaten. Then you become desensitized to insulin --- meaning you don't respond to it --- meaning that your body's natural way to control blood sugar is damaged. And all three of these things lead to craving foods that wreck your health.

    Information about ginger's stabilizing effect came from testing performed in people with Type 2 Diabetes and reported in the 2015 winter edition of the *Iran Journal of Pharmaceutical Research*. Results showed that only 2 grams of powdered ginger taken daily over the course of 12 weeks had the power to dramatically improve blood sugar levels. This is exciting news.

Are you willing to let ginger --- once and for all --- help you stop craving what is bad for you?

Try a green drink with an inch or two of peeled ginger root added and watch and see what happens.

Ginger is a foot soldier in the battle to not overeat.

I do not understand what I do. For what I want to do I do not do, but what I hate I do. (Romans 7:15)

If you struggle with your weight, you know that the battle is constant.

Sometimes it doesn't matter how much you've eaten, you still reach for more. You wonder why. You really don't want to overeat. You really do want to lose weight. You really do want to exercise self-control. You really do want to have leaner muscles and more energy.

But there seems to be something inside that works against you. "For what I want to do I do not do, but what I hate --- I do."

This is why it is so helpful to include in your diet foods that work for you --- foods that help you do what you ought to do. When you've lost the will-power to say no to a second helping or a sugary dessert, ginger can help you get your will-power back. It's reassuring to know that something so small can be used to affect something so big: your self-esteem. Being able to say no to something that's harmful to you strengthens your self-control.

Small amounts of this amazing herb named ginger can help you stop sabotaging your continued attempts to lose those extra pounds --- pounds that have hung around for years.

In 2012 a group of middle-aged, overweight men participated in a study to test the effects of ginger on appetite. Some participants consumed breakfast with --- and others without --- 2 grams of ginger powder dissolved in a hot water beverage. Those who consumed the ginger reported less hunger and, in fact, ate less food than the others.

Researchers concluded (for the benefit of you and me) that ginger could play a role in weight management by causing a person to eat fewer calories, and fewer calories usually mean less weight gain. How helpful it is to know you have a silent warrior working on your behalf to help you reach your weight-loss goal.

Two final benefits:

1. Ginger fights inflammation --- even inflammatory arthritis.

   A controlled trial conducted at the University of Miami in 2001 determined that ginger extract could reduce pain (and the need for other medication) in people who had osteoarthritis of the knee. The study's lead author, Roy Altman, MD, explained that ginger affects specific inflammatory processes at the cellular level.

2. Fresh ginger --- consumed daily --- can even help ease muscle pain caused by exercise.

Have you been feeling any muscle pain from performing any of the movements you've been asked to implement into your day during the last week or so? If so, look to today's goal.

Today's Goal:

Put ginger to the test in today's green drink.

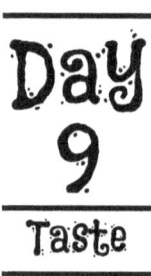

Day 9
Taste

GINGER BLAST GREEN DRINK
(Serves 2)

Ingredients:

- 2 small Granny Smith apples *(peeled if you cannot use organic)*
- 1 large English cucumber *(peeled if you cannot use organic)*
- 4 long leaves dinosaur kale
- 4-5 leaves baby bok choy
- 3 large stalks celery
- 1 small lime *(peeled)*
- 2-inch piece ginger *(peeled, or 1 teaspoon powdered)*
- 1 teaspoon cumin
- 6 English walnut halves

Directions:

- Clean and/or chop: *apples, cucumber, kale, bok choy, celery, lime, & ginger.*
- Put above ingredients --- *except apples* --- through a juicer, then:
- Pour resulting liquid into a blender and add: *apples, cumin, & walnuts.*
- Blend everything together on medium-high speed for 15 seconds, then pour into 2 glasses or glass jars.
- Drink about 1/2 hour before your midday meal.
  (Or refrigerate in a sealed jar for no more than 48 hours.)
- Remember to "chew" each sip.
- Enjoy!

(For the smoothie version, go to www.kriswilliamswellness.com)

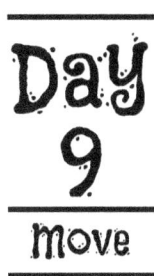

ISOMETRICS FOR YOUR ARMS

While sitting:

Move forward in your chair so that your feet are flat on the floor.

Let your arms hang from your sides.

Grab onto the seat of your chair, one hand on each side of your thighs.

Lean slightly forward,

press into the chair with your arms straightened and tighten the muscles in your arms.

Hold for 5 seconds, then gradually increase to 10.

You might notice that your shoulders have naturally risen.

So next:

Raise your shoulders up to your ears and tighten your shoulder muscles.

Hold for 5 seconds, then gradually increase to 10.

Do each tighten-and-release at least 5 times.

Remember to breathe.

Feel the energy run through your whole body.

Enjoy!

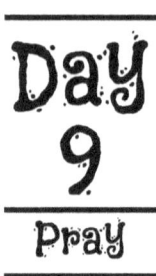

WANTING TO BE WISE

Hello God,

You say that fools despise wisdom.

As far as I know, no one *wants* to be a fool.

I surely don't.

So will you help me always to welcome wise words and wise people into my life?

During this 21-day journey, you know that I'm trying to figure out what the wisest things are for me to eat and drink. And the most prudent way to eat and drink them.

Will you help keep my mind in "search mode" during this journey because it would have never occurred to me to search for help with becoming lean and free using a sometimes forgotten herb like ginger. I never knew ginger could make such a big difference in my weight and health.

Help me to continue to search for wisdom regarding all of the good gifts you offer as if I were searching for gold.

You also say that fools despise discipline.

A strong statement this is...and one that hits a little too close to home.

I admit I've been guilty of ignoring the practice of discipline because, well...

sometimes it appears to take the fun out of life!

And as for discipline regarding food, sometimes it's just too hard to follow through with a balanced eating plan when I'm too tired, too hungry, or too distracted by life's responsibilities.

Please forgive me for allowing myself to ignore discipline.

Please help me know that if I follow your training one day at a time, tolerating discipline will become easier and easier.

I may even come to welcome it.

I *do* want to love both wisdom and discipline…

so I won't be a fool in your eyes…

and so that I might travel further along the road to freedom.

Proverbs 1:7

The fear of the LORD is the beginning of knowledge,
but fools despise wisdom and instruction.

Hebrews 12:11

No discipline seems pleasant at the time,
but painful.
Later on, however,
it produces a harvest of righteousness and peace
for those who have been trained by it.

Day 10
Think

ONE TINY MEDICINE CABINET

Good morning. Glad you're back and able to visit with me again in my herbal garden. There are so many secrets hiding here. So many things you must become mindful of --- if you desire to change your body and your life.

Garlic, for instance. Do you know anything more about it except that it flavors Italian foods and reeks to high heaven?

Would you ever guess that ingesting a daily bulb of smelly garlic could exert a powerful influence on helping you lose weight, maintain your desired weight, or gain more energy?

Garlic is like a tiny (but locked!) medicine cabinet --- full of natural remedies that can bring health and wellness to your body. To access these medicines, you've got to unlock the cabinet. Chopping or crushing a clove of garlic and exposing it to air does the trick. Exposure to oxygen allows a chopped or crushed clove to form sulfur compounds, and it is these sulfur compounds that contain most of garlic's health benefits.

Allicin, one of the compounds formed, is what dispenses garlic's overpowering smell --- which I hope you're willing to ignore --- because allicin is a compound that provides incredible health-giving and weight-controlling properties. *And though heat destroys allicin (a good reason to include raw garlic in your green drinks), other health-giving compounds are formed when heat is applied.*

Before I reveal Garlic's Weight-Loss Secret #10A to you, I need to explain something first. It's about triglycerides. Recognize the word?

They are a type of fat found in your blood. If you have a lot of triglycerides (fat) in your blood, you might be experiencing what doctors call "metabolic syndrome."

Metabolic syndrome is an unhealthy disorder doctors worry about because it manifests five problematic symptoms: high blood pressure, high blood sugar, too much fat around the waist, low HDL cholesterol (the "good" kind), and high triglycerides in your blood.

Garlic's Weight-Loss Secret #10A:

Garlic can help lower triglycerides in your blood.

In 2003, researchers published in the *American Journal of Hypertension* the results of a study which tested the effect allicin would have on fructose-fed rats. (The researchers used a synthetic preparation of allicin to control the dosage.)

Guess what a high-fructose diet produced (See Day 2) in the rats? High blood pressure, high blood sugar, and high triglycerides! And as you would expect, these conditions led to weight gain.

When the fructose-fed rats received allicin, however, their blood pressure, insulin, and triglyceride levels were lowered. Allicin was also shown to prevent further weight gain --- even if the rats continued eating a high-fructose diet.

The rats that didn't receive allicin, however, gained weight.

The researchers recognized the difficulty every dieter has in maintaining a certain weight once pounds are lost, and concluded that allicin is a valuable ingredient for controlling weight.

Garlic's Weight-Loss Secret #10B:

Garlic can help you lose weight.

Another study performed in 2012 examined the effects of aged garlic extract (together with exercise) on cardiovascular disease in 30 Korean women. The findings from this study showed that the women who received 12 weeks of treatment with aged garlic extract (along with a regimen of regular exercise) experienced significant reductions in both body weight and body fat.

Three characteristics of garlic --- its antibacterial, antiviral, and antifungal properties --- make it a useful weight-loss aid because they enable you to stay "over the weather" rather than "under the weather."

Garlic is able to stop an infection from taking over your body because it inhibits the growth of, or even kills, several kinds of dangerous bacteria, including *Staphylococcus* and *Salmonella*. So you can remain dedicated to your weight-loss goals just because you're staying healthy.

Also because of its antibacterial properties, garlic can make sure your waste-removal system is in tip-top shape. One of the first steps to weight-loss is having an efficient elimination system: you've got to be able to rid your body of all the waste produced from processing the food you eat. To eliminate waste, you've got to have good bacteria. A metabolism that lacks good bacteria results in a waste-removal system that's faulty or inefficient --- which results in stubborn weight gain.

Garlic's antibacterial capability helps develop an efficient elimination system because it doesn't kill all the bacteria in your digestive tract (like antibiotics do); it turns out that garlic allows some helpful bacteria ---- like *Lactobacillus acidophilus* --- to continue to grow. When garlic kills off the bad bacteria, good bacteria are able to flourish. Good bacteria are what help breakdown food particles so their waste can be separated and eliminated. Who knew you could win the war on waste removal just by adding a clove or two of garlic to your green drink each day?

Because of garlic's effectiveness in eliminating fungi and harmful yeasts from your system, your ability to remain healthy rises to an entirely different level.

While every single person on the planet is host to some amount of the yeast known as *Candida albicans* (as you saw on Day 5), it's mostly kept under control by the good bacteria in your body. *Candida* sets up house in your small intestines (at first) and is encouraged to grow and multiply by what you feed it: foods high in sugar, simple carbohydrates like refined breakfast cereals, alcohol, white rice and bread, and even pharmaceuticals like corticosteroids, estrogen, birth control pills, and antibiotics. *Candida* growth can even be increased if you have mercury fillings in your teeth.

Candida albicans is able to produce at least 180 chemical toxins --- toxins that remain in your system if you can't control them or excrete them. A few extra colonies of *Candida* might cause you to experience simple unpleasantries like dizziness, offensive body odor, bad breath, frequent bruising, acne, or numbness and tingling in your hands and feet. A bloated stomach ---especially after you eat --- and constipation are two more symptoms. (*Candida albicans* regularly excretes aldehyde, ammonia, and ethanol --- toxins known to cause bloating and constipation.)

But when *Candida* and its by-products have taken over your intestines, you may experience more significant changes, such as hormonal imbalances, PMS, loss of libido, painful intercourse, infertility, insomnia, bronchitis, multiple sclerosis (MS), or Crohn's disease.

If you're still unsure whether or not you have *Candida* overgrowth, try the spit test:

1. *First thing in the morning, before brushing your teeth, fill a clear glass with purified, room-temperature water.*
2. *Gather spit in your mouth (just in your mouth; don't try to cough anything up).*
3. *Spit into the glass of water and watch closely.*
4. *Your saliva will float at first, which is normal.*
5. *Within a few minutes, thin projections that look like hair or small strings may start extending themselves down into the water. If this happens, you may be hosting a Candida party.*
6. *This may take a few minutes, but you don't have to wait longer than fifteen.*

Other positive indications of yeast colonies are:
- *particles that sink slowly and remain suspended in the water*
- *very "cloudy" saliva that sinks to the bottom of the glass within a few minutes.*

If your spit is still floating after about an hour, no worries for you! Your yeast is likely under control.

Garlic's ability to keep fungi and yeasts in check is also a big deal concerning available energy.

When *Candida* flourishes inside of you, it takes away your power --- even your ability to decide what you're going to eat! In fact, one of the ways to recognize if *Candida* has taken over your command center is if you continuously crave sugar and alcohol. You can't get enough of them. (There are other reasons people crave sugar and alcohol, but this is one.)

If you give in to your cravings by packing in a lot of sugar or refined carbohydrates, the cycle starts:

Your blood sugar levels spike. Because you've consumed too much sugar (and/or refined carbs), your body has to work very hard to keep your blood balanced. It does this by rushing insulin to the scene...which causes your blood sugar levels to drop quickly. This causes your brain to automatically believe you need MORE sugar to bring your sugar levels back up again. So you eat more sugar/refined carbs...which causes more insulin to be rushed...

You've experienced this cycle before, and we've talked about it earlier in this guide. It's important to remember --- so you can begin to extricate yourself from this debilitating process.

Candida doesn't just influence *what* you eat...it also keeps making you want *more*... *Candida* is a beast that feeds on large amounts of sugar and starch, and the more it grows, the more it makes you crave foods with large amounts of sugar and starch.

As a result of this ramping-up effect, your hormones get out of whack.

With hormones out of whack, you respond by reaching for whatever food is available (harmful or not) out of disappointment, sadness, or frustration.

And the weight you wanted to lose?

It can't happen.

Except that now you know --- with garlic, it can.

You can break the cycle.

With garlic, you can kill the beast.

You can kill the fungus at its source, and be free to choose.

Choose to blend a clove (or two) of fresh, raw garlic into your green drink today.

Garlic really should be used fresh for most of its health benefits. What's the easiest way to separate the skin from a garlic clove? Place it on a cutting board and pound it with the flat side of a knife. You can use the heel of your hand to do the pounding. This will crush the clove and separate the skins. Cut away the skins and let the crushed clove sit in open air so allicin has a chance to form. After ten minutes the garlic will be ready for you to swallow or add to your juice in a blender. (What you're getting when you use garlic salt is just a lot of sodium, so you should avoid using garlic salt for any benefits.)

You can enjoy the benefits of garlic every day by eating an average-sized clove weighing at least 3 grams.

Concerned about garlic's potent smell? After ingesting fresh garlic:
- chew on a sprig of fresh parsley
- munch on one or two coffee beans
- suck on a slice of lemon
- brush your teeth with baking soda
- have some green tea!

Another option is to use garlic capsules instead of fresh cloves.

Today's Goal:

Go ahead and add a clove of garlic at the blender stage of your green drink!

NOTE: *If taking medications, check with your doctor to see if garlic is compatible with them. Even though garlic is a natural substance, it can still change your body's response to medications or surgery. There's a chance garlic can increase or prolong bleeding and lower blood pressure.*

Day 10
Taste

GARLIC GREEN DRINK
(Serves 2)

Ingredients:

- 2 small Granny Smith apples *(peeled if you cannot use organic)*
- 1 large English cucumber *(peeled if you cannot use organic)*
- 4 long leaves of dinosaur kale
- 4-5 leaves baby bok choy
- 2 large stalks celery
- 1 small lime *(peeled)*
- 2-inch of piece ginger *(peeled, or 1 teaspoon powdered)*
- 2 small cloves garlic *(peeled & smashed 10 minutes before adding to juice)*
- 1 teaspoon of cumin
- 4 Brazil nuts

Directions:

- Clean and/or chop: *apples, cucumber, dinosaur kale, bok choy, celery, lime, & ginger.*
- Put above ingredients --- *except apples* --- through a juicer, then:
- Pour resulting liquid into a blender and add: *apples, garlic, cumin, & Brazil nuts.*
- Blend everything together on medium-high speed for 15 seconds, then pour into 2 glasses or glass jars. *(Refrigerate in sealed jars for no more than 48 hours.)*
- Remember to "chew" each sip.
- Enjoy!

(For the smoothie version, go to www.kriswilliamswellness.com)

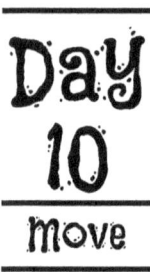

Day 10
move

RISE FROM SITTING
--- at least once every 30 minutes.

When you sit, your anatomy and physiology hover in idle-mode.

Each time you stand up, you rouse your body's muscular system, skeletal system, respiratory system, and circulatory system.

Even a simple movement like standing will go far in energizing you.

Did you know that prolonged sitting has been associated with a larger waist measurement?

The more times you get up from a sitting position, the smaller waistline you can have.

Why not stand up right now to go get a drink of water?

Or:

Instead of sending an email to an office colleague, stand up and take your message in person.

If you're watching TV, stand up when the commercials come on.

Your body will thank you.

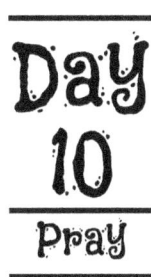

LET ME SEE A CHANGE IN ME

Hello God,

In the Bible you tell the story of Daniel --- the intelligent, young Israelite who, with his three friends, was captured by King Nebuchadnezzar and carried away to live in exile in the pagan city of Babylon.

The story explains that during their indoctrination, Daniel and his friends were required to eat their daily meals from the king's table.

That seemed like a pretty fine arrangement to me. Why wouldn't they have wanted to have their hunger satisfied with any or all of the delicacies and fine foods the kingdom had to offer?

Those foods would have been laid out each day in a tempting array before them, perhaps served with a Babylonian version of a Coca-Cola, Gatorade, or Starbucks Peppermint Mocha Frappuccino Blended Coffee.

But Daniel resisted.

He didn't want to partake of the rich diet the king required. He didn't want to offend you and defile himself with food from the king's table --- knowing that meat and wine from the king's table might have been offered in sacrifice to Babylonian gods.

How did he know that water was one of the secrets to resisting?

Did he know of water's cleansing capability?

Did he know that water could bring life?

Would you help water bring me life, too?

(After ten days of drinking water and eating vegetables, Daniel and his friends looked stronger and healthier than any of the other "recruits" in the program eating from the king's table.)

Will you let me see a change in *me* --- now that I've included drinking water and eating vegetables regularly?

Daniel 1:11-13

Then Daniel said to the steward
whom the chief of the eunuchs had assigned over Daniel,
Hananiah, Mishael, and Azariah,
"Test your servants for ten days;
let us be given vegetables to eat and water to drink.
Then let our appearance and the appearance of the youths
who eat the king's food be observed by you,
and deal with your servants according to what you see."

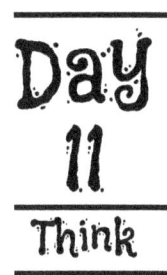

YOUR NUTRIENT FOR SUCCESS

Hi. Though this seems trite, I mean it: Welcome to the first day of the rest of your life.

If you're still struggling to drink a glass of water ---

when you wake up ---

before each meal ---

before each snack---

remember that God's mercies are new every morning. There's hope for success because today you can begin again.

Make a pact with yourself that today you're going to do this.

If you've been drinking water regularly, congratulations! You're halfway there.

You might already have discovered something curious.

You might have made the discovery that when you think you're hungry...what you really are is...thirsty.

We're still visiting in the herb garden, you and I --- because a few more treasures remain buried here --- and I would hate for you to leave before discovering them.

If you are determined to lose weight, maintain your desired weight, or recover your energy, please don't skip learning all you can about this part of the garden. Because its here that you've already found --- and will continue to uncover --- powerful herbs that can make a world of difference in your weight-loss and energy goals.

Like turmeric.

Turmeric is a root herb typically used in Middle Eastern, Northern African, and Southeast Asian cuisine. If you've ever eaten Indian curry, you would have enjoyed turmeric as one of the main ingredients in the spice blends used to flavor it.

But turmeric is much more than a seasoning for curry. The turmeric root houses a powerful substance that could be the solution to every man's and every woman's ill health.

Turmeric could also be one of the best supports for a person struggling with weight-gain.

The compound in turmeric that's believed to be responsible for many of its powerful benefits is called *curcumin*.

Curcumin (not related to another spice called cumin) has been a focus of study most recently because of its antioxidant and anti-inflammatory properties.

We talked about antioxidants on Day 7.

We talked about inflammation before you even began your journey on Day 1, but I'm compelled to discuss it here one more time, because:

Inflammation is always present in the person who holds on to excess pounds that can't be eliminated, in the person who can't maintain his or her weight, and in the person who lacks an adequate amount of energy.

Furthermore, not being able to lose weight, not being able to maintain a healthy weight, and constantly struggling to add more energy all cause stress. And stress causes even more inflammation in your body.

This is a cycle that can lock you in as an anxious prisoner.

You now know that I'm passionate about helping you release yourself from dangerous cycles that lead to ill health and unwanted pounds.

I'm committed to telling you the truth about foods that can work with you to help you lose weight, maintain your weight, and give you the energy you need.

I want to give you hope that after all of your previous attempts, losing weight is possible. Gaining energy is possible.

(I'm also committed to making sure you recognize foods that work against you, too, and you need to be prepared for that! For success in life it's important to know what you shouldn't do, as well as what you should.)

So while you might have to keep your mouth closed to some things, keep your eyes, ears, heart, and mind open to what makes sense and works effectively in your body.

Can this bright orange, gnarly herb really help you lose weight?

Yes!…because it contains curcumin…and…

Curcumin fights inflammation.

With the following added bit of information on inflammation, you'll understand how.

When an organ or structure in your body is inflamed, molecules called *cytokines* go to work. Cytokines stimulate the movement of "healing" cells toward sites of infection, stress, and trauma.

But as you now know, when your structures or organs are continually infected, traumatized, or stressed, healing cells get stimulated over and over again, the sites become crowded with activity, messages get confused, and inflammation never stops. Because inflammation never ends, the infection doesn't heal, trauma and stress don't subside, and damaging processes like insulin resistance and leptin resistance result.

Being able to control (or decrease) the production of cytokines means being able to influence how much or how long your body stays inflamed.

The reason why you don't want to be insulin or leptin resistant is because these two factors are linked to fat gain.

When you are insulin resistant, your body "resists" responding to how much sugar you have in your blood and either makes too little of the insulin hormone, or your body makes too much. Either way, spikes and drops in blood sugar occur.

Here's a brief insulin quiz for you to take right now.

Ask yourself whether you often experience any of these disruptive and damaging symptoms:

- Headaches?
- Bad food cravings?
- Blurred vision?
- Fatigue?
- Nausea?
- Nervousness, shakiness, weakness?
- Dizziness?
- A fast heartbeat and feelings of anxiousness?

If you answer yes to any of these, you may have a resistance to insulin.

When you are leptin resistant, your brain "resists" responding to leptin (the hormone that tells your brain you've had enough to eat). When leptin isn't functioning, you have trouble recognizing when you're "full" after a meal or after a snack, so you keep on eating.

Here's a brief leptin quiz for you to take right now. There are only two questions:

1. Do you open a bag of chips or cookies and polish off the whole thing, even though you're not really hungry?
2. Do you finish whatever foods you have on your plate (no matter how large the portions are), just because they're there, and you feel stuffed when you're done?

If you answered yes to either of these two questions, you might be leptin resistant.

But here's the good news: *curcumin has been shown to decrease levels of insulin and leptin resistance, even and especially in a high-fat diet.*

Curcumin detoxifies your liver.

Fat burning is critical for weight-loss, and your liver is the organ that's critical for fat burning. Studies have found that when the liver gets damaged, detoxification decreases, and weight-loss doesn't happen.

Curcumin fights cancer.

Many health professionals recommend using curcumin regularly, not only for weight-loss but also because it has also been shown to mitigate the effect of other food components that are known to cause cancer. (As long as you're losing weight, why wouldn't you want to be fighting cancer, too?)

Consider curcumin your success nutrient!

Curcumin can stop you from regaining the weight you've worked so hard to lose.

This is one big, final reason to include curcumin in your diet.

A person typically gains weight because fat tissues grow and expand through the formation of new blood vessels. In 2009, a study performed at Tufts University found that curcumin actually suppressed fat-tissue growth in mice. Mice fed curcumin were unable to form new blood vessels (and the growth and increase in fat cells can't happen without new blood vessels). They were found to have less fat gain than those who did not consume the curcumin antioxidant, even though both groups were eating high-fat diets.

Now you might be thinking, "Curcumin works with rats, but what about with people? What about me? Will curcumin really work for me?" So I'm excited to share with you the results of a more recent study that was conducted in 2015 on people.

Researchers stated that their findings suggest that a bioavailable form of curcumin can positively influence weight management in overweight people.

What are bioavailable forms of curcumin?

If you want curcumin to be effective as you travel along with this Think, Taste, Move, & Pray Guide, it's not enough to merely add raw or powdered turmeric/curcumin to your food or drink according to taste.

The reasons why are these:

The amount of curcumin in a turmeric root is a meager 3%.

If you eat it raw, your body absorbs only about one percent because any kind of curcumin is poorly absorbed by the body.

Here are some recommended methods to help your body more readily absorb curcumin (or make it bioavailable):

- Add black pepper to your food or juice at the same time you add turmeric/curcumin.
- Take a turmeric/curcumin supplement with at least 95 percent curcuminoids. (Each capsule should contain 400-600 mg of curcumin. You can take one of these capsules three times a day, or as directed on the label. Look for products that contain bioperine or piperine, which are black pepper extracts that increase curcumin's bioavailability by 2000 %.)
- Consume turmeric/curcumin with beneficial fats. Curcumin is fat-soluble, so you're going to need a bit of coconut oil, olive oil, or avocado to help dissolve this magical compound. Or as I suggest in today's drink: add nuts to your curcumin-flavored green drink.
- Eat turmeric/curcumin with quercetin.
  Quercetin is a plant pigment known as a "flavonoid" (a type of polyphenol --- or micronutrient --- with antioxidant capability found most abundantly in whole foods) which also helps to significantly increase the activity of curcumin. So if you want to make sure curcumin does its work without interference, eat it along with foods high in quercetin: apples, cranberries, blueberries, raw kale, red leaf lettuce, fresh broccoli, fresh spinach, onions, and red wine. You might already be including quercetin if you are drinking green tea --- which I offered you a cup of on Day 4.

Many of these ingredients above will fit well into a delicious green juice or smoothie. Start with the juice recipe on today's Taste menu. Then, as you get comfortable, add different vegetables and --- go ahead --- shake in some turmeric/curcumin (with pepper)!

A simple, convenient, and perhaps best method of consuming curcumin for achieving clinical results is to take curcumin in supplement form. Choose a high-quality turmeric extract that contains 100 percent certified organic ingredients, with at least 95 percent curcuminoids.

If you want anti-inflammatory results, you need to get 500 to 1,000 milligrams of curcuminoids per day. If you're using freshly-ground turmeric, figure that there are about 200 milligrams of curcumin in one teaspoon (though the amount varies depending on the source and growing conditions).

Today's Goal:

Add turmeric/curcumin and black pepper at the blender stage of your green drink.

Check for beneficial brands of turmeric/curcumin at: *www.kriswilliamswellness.com.*

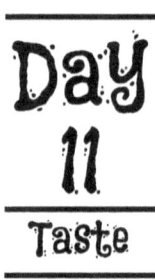

Day 11 — Taste

SALAD AS JUICE
(Serves 2)

Ingredients:

- 2 small Granny Smith apples *(peeled if you cannot use organic)*
- 1 large English cucumber *(peeled if you cannot use organic)*
- ½ head red leaf lettuce
- 5-6 leaves romaine lettuce
- 6-8 large dandelion greens
- 3 large stalks celery
- 1 lime *(peeled)*
- 2-inch piece ginger *(peeled, or 1 teaspoon powdered)*
- 2 small cloves garlic *(smashed & peeled 10 minutes ahead)*
- 1 tablespoon ground turmeric/curcumin
- ½ teaspoon black pepper
- 2 tablespoons pine nuts

Directions:

- Clean and/or chop: *apples, cucumber, red leaf lettuce, romaine lettuce, dandelion greens, celery, lime, & ginger.*
- Put above ingredients --- *except apples* --- through a juicer, then:
- Pour resulting liquid into a blender & add: *apples, garlic, turmeric, black pepper, & pine nuts.*
- Blend on medium-high speed for 15 seconds, then pour into 2 glasses or glass jars.
- *Refrigerate in sealed jars for no more than 48 hours.*
- Remember to "chew" each sip, and enjoy!

(For the smoothie version, go to www.kriswilliamswellness.com)

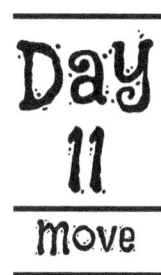

TOUCH YOUR TOES

Stand with your feet hip-width apart.

Breathe in.

Breathe out and bend over with your arms and hands straight down.

Keep your legs straight, *but don't lock your knees.*

Touch your toes *(or reach down as far as you can)*.

Come back to a straight-standing position.

Repeat touching your toes and then straightening to a standing position 10 times.

Next:

Stand with your feet one foot out from each side of your hip (at least 2 ½ feet apart) --- in a wide V position.

Stretch your arms out to your sides.

Bend at the waist and --- while keeping your legs straight *(but without locking your knees)* --- try to touch your right hand to your left foot.

Come back up to an upright position and reposition arms out to your sides.

Next:

Bend at your waist and try to touch your left hand to your right foot.

Come back up to an upright position and reposition arms out

to your sides so that you can repeat the bends and alternate hand-to-foot touches 10 times on each side.

Each day you do this you'll be able to stretch further.

Rejoice when you can wrap your fingers around your toes while keeping your legs straight *(without locking your knees)*.

Enjoy the energy you feel!

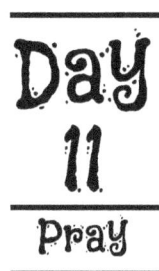

WANTING TO BE HEALTHY

Hello God,

Help me to recognize that I don't have all the answers.

Help me not to be wise in my own eyes.

Help me to be willing to compare what I think I "know"

with information that is tested, well-researched, and respected.

And help me to turn away from things that harm me ---

or offend you.

Proverbs 3: 7-8

Do not be wise in your own eyes;
fear the Lord and shun evil.
This will bring health to your body
and nourishment to your bones.

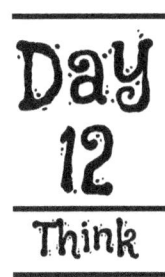

GIVING UP...AND STARTING OVER

Diet books told you that to lose weight you had to restrict the number of calories you ate.

You tried that. You lost a few pounds, but then your weight wouldn't budge.

Friends told you that you must have been eating more than you thought you were (even though you felt like you were eating just enough to survive).

And so you carefully counted, measured, restricted. Still your weight plateaued.

You didn't know what to do. How could you decrease the number of calories you were eating any more than you already had?

The temptation to revert to eating all of your "favorite foods" that you'd been denying yourself was too strong to resist. So you gave up and gave in.

What was the point, anyway?

Isn't life to enjoy?

...

Of course it is!

And surely what makes it less enjoyable is trying to lose weight by denying yourself "favorite foods" over and over again. What makes it depressing is making that kind of sacrifice and still getting stuck at a certain weight!

Because you are one who might have been bewildered by this experience, I'd like to ask you to consider two concepts:

1. How "favorite foods" become favorites.
2. Why a dieter's weight won't budge.

Foods become favorites in a couple of ways.

Early in our journey together we talked about the addictive nature of sugar. So you can now understand that foods containing sugar may have become your "favorites" simply because...you're addicted to them. You can't resist them. In fact, you're a slave to them. (Hopefully, by now you've been willing to try some of the ways offered in this guide to free yourself from this addiction?)

A second reason foods may have become your favorites is because you've eaten them since childhood. You're accustomed to their smells, textures, and flavors. They're your favorites just because you're in the habit of eating them.

But just because you're in the habit of eating something doesn't mean it's healthy for you. And just because unhealthy foods *have been* your favorites doesn't mean you can't get used to eating healthy foods and *make them your favorites now*. If you begin to make healthy foods your favorites, then they'll be the ones you'll choose when you're tired, hungry, depressed, or stressed.

Would you be willing to consider the possibility of forming this new habit?

A habit is formed by doing the same thing over and over again. Whether good or bad --- because of repetition --- that habit plants sturdy roots in your subconscious being.

If you've spent years giving in to the habit of choosing foods that destroy your health, I want to caution you that your will and your spirit will resist as you try to change your food choices. But you can practice the habit of making healthy choices. If you at first don't like a food that brings life to you --- a certain fruit or vegetable, for example --- you can come to like it if you eat it often enough. And picture this: if you once dieted by restricting calories and then gave up and gave in, what would have happened if the "favorite foods" you wanted to return to for comfort were all the foods that give you health and vitality?

You picked up this book because your spirit is crying out to be free.

To weaken and destroy destructive habits you've got to grow new roots --- roots that will anchor you and sustain you when the temptations to revert to old, unhealthy ways of eating come like a storm.

God wants to give you hope that it can be done. You can grow new roots.

Will you trust Him to help you? Will you take Him at His word? He wants you to experience the beauty of self-control. He wants you to experience the freedom that discipline brings.

He says that those who hope in Him will renew their strength. "They will soar on wings like eagles; they will run and not grow weary, they will walk and not be faint." (Isaiah 40:31)

How can you change an unhealthy habit that has you under its power?

One of the first things to do is to trust that the Lord is with you, fighting at your side. He's with you, He says, if you take Him as your God. He doesn't want you to be dismayed but promises to strengthen you and help you. "I will uphold you with my righteous right hand," He promises (Isaiah 41:10).

A second thing to do is to consider this question:

What would it look like if you tasted a new healthy food *at least twelve different times* --- to see if it could become a favorite? Eating by experimenting could begin a new habit that would lead you in the direction of becoming lean and free.

Now as to your weight plateauing: is it just your imagination, or can it really happen?

It really can happen.

Trying to lose weight by limiting calories does make your weight plateau --- because limiting calories decreases the speed of your metabolism. And the speed of your metabolism is one key to how many calories you burn.

You should know that the One who created you provided ways to solve this conundrum.

One solution is to increase your body's metabolic rate. New evidence shows that cayenne pepper (made from dried chili powder) may help counteract the decrease in metabolic rate that often occurs during weight-loss.

Cayenne pepper is effective because it contains a powerful little ingredient known as *capsaicin*.

Capsaicin is the compound that gives pepper its spicy hot taste. Capsaicin is also the compound that's responsible for thermogenesis, a process that creates heat in your body. Thermogenesis is a good thing when you're trying to lose weight because it promotes three biological activities:

- It speeds up your metabolism.
- It helps decrease your appetite.
- It helps fight fat buildup.

Research has proven that consuming thermogenic ingredients ---like cayenne, chili, and habanero peppers --- can boost your metabolism, possibly by up to 5 percent, and increase fat burning by up to 16 percent.

A study conducted at Purdue University in 2010 showed that peppers decreased appetite, especially in people who said they didn't usually eat spicy foods.

(People who didn't like eating spicy foods had better weight-loss results when they started taking cayenne capsules.)

This same study found that after adding about half a teaspoon of cayenne pepper --- either mixed in food or swallowed in a capsule --- normal-weight young adults ate 60 fewer calories at their next meal AND burned an extra 10 calories. (If this seems like a small amount to you, consider what consuming-fewer-calories + extra-calories-burned add up to over time!)

Not only does capsaicin speed up your metabolism and burn more calories, it also targets the places on your body where it burns fat first. Scientific reviews by food-scientist Stephen Whiting at

Manchester Metropolitan University in Manchester, England, showed that capsaicin triggers an adrenalin rush. And it's the adrenalin rush that specifically orders your brain to burn fat cells.

Dr. Whiting's research found that fat around the belly was burned most rapidly. This is the fat that's most dangerous, and this is the fat you're probably most concerned about.

Now if you begin to take capsaicin regularly, you need to be aware that as your body becomes more accustomed to the hot spice, more capsaicin will be required to raise your body temperature and create the same fat-burning effect.

When you add cayenne pepper to your diet for weight-loss, the results might be subtle at first.

But don't give up.

Eat colorful spicy foods, and enjoy what you eat!

Today's Goal:

Shake some cayenne pepper into your carrot drink.

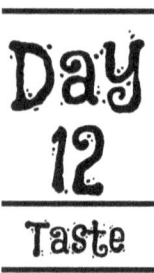

Day 12
Taste

CELEBRATING CARROTS DRINK
(Serves 2)

Ingredients:

1 large English cucumber
6 medium-sized organic carrots *(no need to peel; just clean & trim away tops & toes)*
1 small beet
4 stalks celery
2-inch piece ginger *(peeled or 1 teaspoon powdered)*
1 lime *(peeled)*
1 Granny Smith apple
2 small cloves garlic *(peeled & smashed 10 minutes ahead)*
1 tablespoon turmeric/curcumin
½ teaspoon black pepper
cayenne pepper *(start with a pinch, & gradually increase amount)*
6 English walnuts

Directions:

- Clean and/or chop: *cucumber, carrots, beet, celery, & lime.*
- Put all above ingredients through a juicer first, then:
- Pour liquid into a blender & add: *apple, garlic, turmeric, cayenne pepper, black pepper, & walnuts.*
- Blend for 15 seconds, then pour into 2 glasses or glass jars.
- *Refrigerate in sealed jars for no more than 48 hours.*
- Remember to "chew" each sip.
- Enjoy!

(For the smoothie version, go to www.kriswilliamswellness.com)

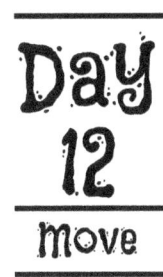

TAKE A 12 MINUTE WALK

It doesn't matter to where.

You can walk around your house, in the hallway of your apartment building, or to the corner store.

If you enjoy the scenery when you walk, you'll be inclined to walk again.

When you walk, walk with intention. Step forward with your right foot as far as you can, heel first.

Then step forward with your left foot as far as you can, heel first.

When you walk, allow your arms to swing freely from your sides.

Let your left arm swing forward while your right foot is stepping forward.

Then let your right arm swing forward while your left foot is stepping forward.

Find your rhythm. Breathe in. Breathe out.

Enjoy!

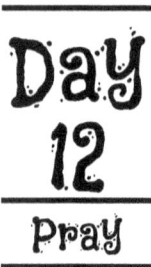

Day 12
Pray

PLEASE PUT A WALL OF PROTECTION AROUND ME

Hello God,

I'm beginning to understand that what I listen to, what I pay attention to, the thoughts I mull over inside my head, can affect my health just as much as what I eat.

I want to be able to guard my mind, my will, and my emotions as you ask me to.

Will you help me filter out, then, any thoughts that lead me down paths to emotional and spiritual destruction?

Will you help me refuse any thoughts that lead me down paths to low energy and physical illness?

Will you help me now to think about the possibility of enjoying foods that are good for me...instead of turning up my nose at them?

Will you give me the desire (from my heart) to be willing to try them?

Will you help me to understand that if I eat foods that are good for me, I can teach my body to like them --- even to crave them --- if I try them at least twelve times. Some call this the "wisdom of the body." And you're the One who made my body very smart, smart enough to crave what's good for it if I give it a chance.

Proverbs 4: 20-23

My son, pay attention to what I say;
turn your ear to my words.
Do not let them out of your sight,
keep them within your heart;
for they are life to those who find them
and health to one's whole body.
Above all else, guard your heart,
for everything you do flows from it.

Day 13
Think

GARDEN DELIGHTS

Good morning! So glad you're still here with me in the garden! I hope you now realize that in this immense world of ours, there are a thousand and one herbs and spices for you to take advantage of...a thousand and one more ways that your God and creator has provided for you to add variety to the things you eat...a thousand and one more possibilities to not only make your foods more interesting and flavorful but also healthier to eat.

The herbs I've shared with you on Days 9, 10, 11, and 12 will keep you "gassed up" as you travel on the road to good health and healthy weight-loss.

Still, there's one more spice you're absolutely going to want to know about before we wander back inside.

It's one final spice included in your 21-Day Exploratory Guide for weight-loss and energy.

So let me introduce you to *cinnamon*.

I know you already recognize it by its smell.

And if you're like me, whenever you smell it, you're tricked into thinking there's a sugary treat on the way.

But cinnamon doesn't only have to be associated with "expensive" foods --- foods that are loaded with sugar or refined carbohydrates --- foods that can cause weight gain and cost you your health.

Cinnamon can also be associated with health and healthy weight-loss.

From this point forward let cinnamon have these new associations for you.

Cinnamon is a powerful weapon to assist you in the battle to lose weight, maintain your desired weight, and restore to you the energy you need because of its following capabilities:

- **Cinnamon provides a regulating effect on sugar levels in your blood by increasing your insulin levels.**
  You now know that regulating sugar levels is vital for weight-loss and overall health because when there's no regulation, addictive behavior sets in. You become unable to resist junk-food cravings. You become controlled by frequent mood swings. Junk-food cravings mean you reach for "expensive" foods that keep the cycle spinning and leave you eating the wrong things. And frequent mood swings mean you're probably eating not because you're hungry, but because you're depressed, stressed, or fatigued.

  Regulating blood sugar levels and simultaneously increasing insulin availability prevent the onset of that terribly disruptive syndrome called Metabolic Syndrome --- the one that leads to further weight-gain and obesity. Cinnamon is an effective blood regulator because it contains plant nutrients (polyphenols) and the mineral chromium which help improve how your body uses insulin.

  How much cinnamon do you need to help control blood sugar levels? James A. Duke, Ph.D., a botanist and author of The CRC Handbook of Medicinal Herbs, says ½ to ¾ teaspoon of ground cinnamon daily is enough. And only one-eighth of a teaspoon of cinnamon will triple your insulin efficiency.

- **Cinnamon increases your metabolism (the speed your body uses to perform all of its functions).**
  You already understand that if you've got a lot of glucose/sugar passing through your blood, your body automatically knows it's supposed to store what you don't immediately use. Sugar is stored as fat (which is energy in reserve for later use). If your metabolism increases, you need more glucose/sugar for the boosted energy requirements ---

which leaves less glucose/sugar to be sent to your liver for storage. Cinnamon intake = increased metabolism = less fat storage = less weight on your body!

- ***Cinnamon improves your gut health...***
because it's a powerful "cleansing" agent for your digestive tract. A component in cinnamon --- called *trans-Cinnamaldehyde* --- is capable of getting rid of a particular type of bacteria known as *Clostridium difficile*. It's this bacteria which various studies show to be instrumental in weight gain.

- ***Cinnamon controls the growth of Candida albicans.***
As you read on Day 10, *Candida albicans* takes away your power to lose weight or maintain a healthy weight. The Candida yeast affects the balance of bacteria in your gut, slows down your metabolism, and disrupts how your body gets rid of waste. If you can't get rid of waste, you can't get rid of weight.

- ***Cinnamon lengthens the time it takes for food to pass from your stomach into your intestines.***
The result? You feel satisfied for a more extended period of time, and you don't go back to the refrigerator for more food an hour after you've just eaten. In one study, after 14 healthy subjects were served 1.5 cups (300 grams) of plain rice pudding, researchers measured how quickly the subjects' stomachs emptied. Subsequently, these same subjects were served 1.5 cups (300 grams) of rice pudding flavored with 1.2 teaspoons (6 grams) of cinnamon. After eating the cinnamon pudding, the researchers found that the subjects had a lower rate of emptying (34.5%) compared to when they had eaten the plain pudding (37%). But most importantly, the cinnamon had significantly lessened the rise in blood sugar levels after its consumption.

Nevertheless, even though cinnamon may prevent more fat from being added to your body and may help you feel satisfied longer, cinnamon will contribute very little to losing or maintaining your weight if you continue to remain…immobile. That is, and I say this gently, my friend, if you don't do any kind of movement or exercise, and if the majority of the foods you eat consist of fast and processed foods, you won't lose weight even if you consume huge amounts of cinnamon.

But if you're willing to change…even little by little…you'll see results.

What you must also be aware of is this: *consuming very high levels of cinnamon could be dangerous. Safety depends on what type of cinnamon you ingest and how much.*

There are 2 varieties of cinnamon --- for flavoring both sweet and savory dishes ---that are available in the marketplace today: **Cassia cinnamon**, produced in China, Vietnam, and Indonesia; and **Ceylon cinnamon** (also known as "true" cinnamon) produced in Sri Lanka, India, Madagascar, Brazil, and the Caribbean.

What you probably find in your grocery store is cassia cinnamon, because it is more readily available and cheaper than Ceylon cinnamon.

The more critical issues are whether both cassia and Ceylon have the same medicinal properties, and whether both are equally safe.

Most of the research showing that cinnamon can lower blood sugar has utilized cassia cinnamon (although more research is being performed with Ceylon cinnamon, and the results are comparable).

But cassia cinnamon from China, Vietnam and Indonesia contains a relatively high amount of a substance called coumarin, and when cassia is consumed in large portions, coumarin can cause liver damage in susceptible people. Studies in rats and mice have also found that coumarin consumed in very large doses over long periods of time did provoke cancer (although there is no evidence it does the same for humans). While the effects appear to be reversible, the danger is undeniable, so it's important to pay attention to the type of cinnamon you consume, especially if you consume high amounts over a long period of time.

Cassia cinnamon contains approximately 200 times (about 8% by volume) more coumarin than Ceylon cinnamon, which contains only 0.04% of coumarin by volume.

Conversely, Ceylon cinnamon contains higher levels of cinnamon oil than cassia, and it's the oil in which the majority of cinnamon's medicinal properties are found. So if you intend to use cinnamon for weight-loss, it is recommended that you use Ceylon cinnamon.

How much cinnamon is safe to consume?

According to the US National Health Service, you should not take more than one teaspoon (5g) of cinnamon per day for more than six weeks at a time. You could, for instance, take it for five days, rest for two days, and then repeat the cycle. Since Ceylon cinnamon contains very little coumarin, you can usually double this dosage --- which means you can safely take up to 2 teaspoons of Ceylon cinnamon a day.

Monitoring your intake is possible with supplements, but (remarkably!) not all supplements have their coumarin content labeled. To be safe, why not use Ceylon cinnamon even if you're using just one teaspoon of cinnamon a day?

One easy way to include cinnamon as you travel through food country:

Make cinnamon tea by adding 1/4 teaspoon of ground cinnamon (or use up to 2 cinnamon sticks) to 1 1/2 cups of boiled (filtered or spring) water. Let sit for 2 or 3 minutes. Pour the liquid through a coffee filter to separate out the undissolved powder, and transfer the brew into a cup.

When are the best times to drink this tea? On an empty stomach, or before bed.

You can also dust cinnamon over fruits like blueberries, apples, apple sauce, and bananas.

I like sprinkling about a half teaspoon over sprouted-protein or gluten-free bread that I've coated with almond butter. (And if I haven't gone over my 15 grams of fructose for the day, I'll drizzle some raw honey over the bread, too.)

You can also add cinnamon to:

- your morning apple cider vinegar drink
- coconut milk
- almond milk
- coffee

Are you sold on cinnamon and ready to use it as a weight-loss aid? Please consult your doctor if you're using medications. (*Remember: both types of cinnamon contain some amount of coumarin, a natural blood-thinner, and this may interfere with your medications.*)

Please consult your doctor if you're pregnant or nursing.

Please don't offer high doses to children.

Consult a health professional if you decide to use cinnamon tablets or pills for weight-loss. The truth is, they can be effective if you take no more than 2000 mg of cinnamon a day --- and if you make sure the type of cinnamon in the pills or tablets is Ceylon cinnamon.

Choose 500 mg pills so you can take 2000 mg throughout the day.

Take 1 pill in the morning, 2 at midday, and the final one with your evening meal.

Also understand that taking cinnamon in excess can suppress your central nervous system and have a toxic effect on your liver.

Excess amounts might also cause sores in your mouth and inflammation of your tongue, stomach intestines, skin, mucous membranes or urinary tract.

If you experience dizziness, drowsiness, vomiting or diarrhea after taking cinnamon for a while, you'll know you've taken too much.

Today's Goal:

Add at least 1/4 teaspoon of ground cinnamon to one of your favorite drinks, fruits, or foods.

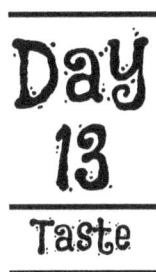

SIMPLE CINNAMON SMOOTHIE
(Serves 2)

Ingredients:

1 cup frozen blueberries
¼ cup frozen cherries *(6-8 cherries, without pits)*
4-inch piece banana *(fresh or frozen)*
1 ½ cup purified water
2 teaspoons Ceylon cinnamon

Directions:

- Put all of the above ingredients into a blender, then blend on medium-to-high for 15-20 seconds.
- Pour into 2 glasses or glass jars.
- Remember to chew each mouthful of your smoothie.
- Enjoy! (Believe me, you will!)

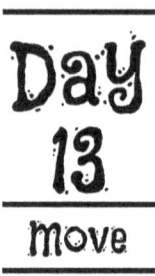

Day 13
move

PARK FARTHER AWAY…

from the entrance to your home, apartment building, office building, shopping center, or grocery store.

Practice the release walk you just did yesterday.

If you carry a purse or bag, see if you can get one that straps across your body so your arms are free to swing and you can walk with abandon.

Feel the energy run through your whole body.

Enjoy the fact that you've given a gift to someone else: that empty parking spot nearer the entrance to the place where you're going.

Go ahead and smile at your own generosity.

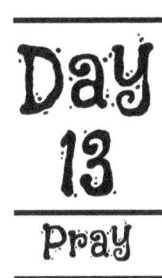

VARIETY: THE SPICE OF LIFE

Hello God,

During these past few "miles" of my journey, I've learned about an assortment of spices you created so that the flavors of foods can be enhanced.

And I marvel at how, by using them, I can access multiple ways to succeed in becoming lean, healthy, and free.

Who would have ever thought that herbs and spices could entice me to eat healthy foods that I'm not yet used to eating or have avoided in the past?

Who would have ever thought that so many "magical" elements that enhance health could be found in the herbs and spices themselves?

I want to use everything you've provided on this earth to enable me to succeed in my weight management goals. So from today on, help me to find inventive ways to include in my diet as many seasonings as you've created for me to enjoy.

Will you prod me to make a plan for hunting and gathering all those food "flavors" that are good for me?

I'm thinking that preparing a meal using herbs I've never before experimented with might be an enjoyable challenge.

Who could I invite to share this meal with me?

Proverbs 31: 10-14

A wife of noble character who can find?
... She is like the merchant ships,
bringing her food from afar.

Hebrews 13:16

And do not forget to do good and to share with others,
for with such sacrifices God is pleased.

John 21: 9-12

When they landed,
they saw a fire of burning coals there with fish on it, and some bread.
Jesus said to them, "Bring some of the fish you have just caught."
So Simon Peter climbed back into the boat and dragged the net ashore.
It was full of large fish, 153, but even with so many the net was not torn.
Jesus said to them, "Come and have breakfast."

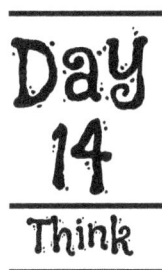

PARTY FIBER

You've been doing a lot of drinking for the last thirteen days, and I hope that you've gotten just a little bit drunk...on all things valuable for you:

- fresh, filtered or spring water
- apple cider vinegar
- teas
- blended fruits
- green juices

Nevertheless, I'm sure you've still been wondering when we were going to get around to talking about meals...meals that are composed of the kind of foods you chew. Meals that you can actually, well, eat. Meals that are easy to prepare, enjoyable, good for you, and NOT EXPENSIVE.

Remember when we spoke before about EXPENSIVE foods?

EXPENSIVE foods are foods to avoid --- they are the extra-sweet and processed foods that are full of added sugar, HFCS, and other refined carbohydrates --- foods that add excessive pounds to your body and cost you your health.

We've also talked about FREE foods --- the kind of foods that give you nutrients your body can use and the kinds of foods you can eat as much of as you want.

FREE foods are the kind of foods that happen to help you lose weight, maintain your weight, and have more energy, too. They do this not just because they're low in calories, but also because they're the kind of foods you have to chew.

And chewing is crucial for your health. Yes, chewing!

Chewing is even crucial for healthy weight-loss.

Eating foods that you have to chew doesn't mean you do all that work for nothing. You get the following rewards:

- Having to chew slows your pace, preventing you from easily gulping down mega-calories. (For instance, you can "inhale" a Hostess Twinkie with little-to-no chewing, but you can't "inhale" a raw carrot.)
- Having to chew helps you become mindful. You can't talk while you're chewing (or at least you shouldn't!) and so you focus on the food in front of you. When you're mindful, you tend to breathe more deeply, and as a result, your digestion works more smoothly.
- Having to chew helps you truly taste (and enjoy) each morsel. If you linger to enjoy each bite, you tend to take fewer mouthfuls, because you have time to recognize when you are full or satisfied.
- Having to chew fibrous foods means you're eating foods that provide your body with an essential ingredient.

Would you believe that all of the above benefits actually help you lose weight, maintain your weight, and provide energy?

I kid you not.

Let's talk about the last benefit.

Does your body really need fiber, and will it actually help you lose weight?

Of course you've already guessed that the answer is "yes" to both questions.

Fiber --- both digestible and indigestible --- is the part of each carbohydrate that requires chewing. The fiber in foods like whole grains and seeds is contained in the bran or the coat of the seed. The fiber in fruits and vegetables is provided in the parts that are not the juice.

Fiber is useful for you because it provides bulk for your digestive tract, and bulk increases peristaltic action in your digestive tract. Peristaltic action is the wave-like motion in your stomach and intestines that helps move food particles through your system and waste particles out of it so that you can have regular bowel movements. If you are regular, your body is repeatedly getting rid of metabolic waste and toxins, leaving you feeling healthier and more energetic.

How much fiber do you need to include in your diet each day to prevent constipation and maintain insulin health?

If you're a man between 18 and 50 years old, your body needs between 30 and 50 grams a day; if you're a man over 50, you could get by with a little less --- but no less than 30 grams. If you're a woman between 18 and 50 years old, your body needs at least 25 grams a day. If you're a woman 51 years old and older, your body needs about 21 grams a day.

Another way to measure: make sure you consume 14 grams of fiber for every 1,000 calories in your diet.

In regards to weight-loss, when you are regular in your bowel movements, you naturally have fewer mood-swings and as a result, are less likely to overeat. Fibrous foods are also less likely to cause you to become depressed or anxious.

A study published in the February 17, 2015 edition of *Annals of Internal Medicine* suggests that it's possible to concentrate on only one thing to lose weight: aim to eat the amount of fiber recommended to you in your age group above. (Or, include at least 14 grams for every 1,000 calories you consume.) If you do this one simple thing, you can lose weight. (Participants in studies conducted lost 4 ½ pounds in 12 weeks.) Are you willing to try it for yourself?

Fiber can also help you maintain your desired weight. If you're wondering right now if there's an uncomplicated way to include fiber in your meals and snacks, you know that I'm going to tell you there is.

Let's talk first about seeing if we can put some fiber back into your drinks.

Hopefully during these past thirteen days, when you've added fruits to any of your green juices, you've blended the fruits in a blender first (as I suggested), so that you ended up consuming the whole fruits --- both juice and fiber.

If you've been using a juicer for your greens during these past thirteen days, you've been extracting the plant juices from their fibers and (perhaps) throwing the fiber away.

That's just what I did when I started. I decided not to use my blender for green veggies (at first) because juice made in a blender using all parts of the fruits and vegetables was too thick for me, and I didn't like the taste.

So I understand if you've been doing the same thing, and I don't want you to worry. All is well. Everything in time. Eventually, you may want to make all parts of your juice in a blender, as I do now.

Because then you, like me, would be consuming in your green juice much of the fiber your body needs each day. Until then, I'm going to share with you a simple way to add fiber to drinks made in a juicer.

And the secret about this fiber is that it will also help you lose weight. The fiber I'm talking about is contained in a unique seed: flaxseed.

The fiber in flaxseed is mucilaginous, meaning that it can absorb fluid and expand. A small amount will help you feel "full" and satisfied, and these feelings should prevent you from eating more food than your body needs.

1 tablespoon of flaxseed will give you about 2 grams of fiber, so consuming 2 to 4 tablespoons will *start* you on fulfilling your fiber needs for the day. If your fiber intake has been very low up until now, start with one tablespoon --- to prevent digestion discomfort --- and you probably shouldn't include more than 5 tablespoons a day. (Can you guess how many grams of fiber most people eat in total each day? Answer: 11 grams, or only one half --- or less --- of what's needed!)

The lignans in flaxseed are plant estrogens that may help you reach your weight-loss goals by keeping you regular. If you don't have frequent bowel movements (for most people this means excreting waste at least once a day), your body is probably holding onto toxic substances that are slowly destroying its structural integrity. By eating whole ground flaxseed, dangerous waste (that forms poisonous substances) is expelled from your body more frequently.

Lignans can help you reach your weight-loss goals by decreasing your chances of experiencing metabolic syndrome. They work by lowering fat and glucose levels in your blood, and as long as you don't continue to over-eat, lignans will help get you to your right weight.

The omega-3 fatty acids in flaxseed may also facilitate dropping some extra pounds.

Omega-3 fatty acids are a type of fat known to feed your brain, making it feel "happy." Omega-3s send signals to your cerebral gray matter that you are full, that you've received an adequate amount of calories and nutrients, and that you don't need to eat for a while.

Maybe you've been on diets that allowed only low-fat foods, and you continued to be hungry all day long. When you didn't feel satisfied, you probably "cheated" your way out of the diet a lot of the time. And this conduct probably made you (and your body) feel like the task of losing weight was and is hopeless.

On the other hand, maybe your daily routine at the moment has you eating fast-food burgers, fries, vegetable-oil pizzas and doughnuts --- all foods filled with harmful and very "unhappy" fats --- so you still haven't been feeling full or satisfied with what would be a "normal" portion. You end up eating more than you should of these foods, and this conduct probably makes you (and your body) feel like a failure.

If you've allowed yourself to become ensnared by either of these behaviors, do not fear! You can "unset" the traps!

Flaxseed, with its fiber, lignans, and omega-3 poly-unsaturated fats will help you feel full, content, clean, and in control.

Ways to include flaxseed in your day:

- Spoon 1 to 3 tablespoons of ground flaxseeds into your morning juice.
- Sprinkle ground seeds into your Greek yogurt, bowl of soup, or lunch or dinner salad.

One tablespoon of ground flaxseed contains 37 calories. (A standard serving is 2 tablespoons per 100 pounds of body weight. Calories in a serving: 74.)

Make sure you drink plenty of fluids when you are taking flax so that you don't end up constipated. (Drink at least 4 ounces for every tablespoon of ground flaxseed.)

The best way to buy flaxseeds is to buy them whole, protect them in a glass jar in the refrigerator, and then grind them as you need them. Because flaxseeds go rancid quickly after grinding, it is a good idea to eat them right away or store the pulverized portion in the refrigerator, making sure you eat the flaxseed "flour" within a day or two. (And you should grind flaxseeds before eating them, by the way, because whole seeds would just pass right through your system without your receiving the benefit of their nutrients.)

Some brands advertise "cold-milling" --- a commercial-grinding process which promises to retain the integrity of the fats for months at a time after the seeds have been ground...But, I'd still suggest buying fresh and grinding fresh.

Today's Goal:

Include at least one tablespoon of freshly ground flaxseed in your juice, smoothie, soup, yogurt or salad. Add up to three tablespoons a day as your body adjusts.

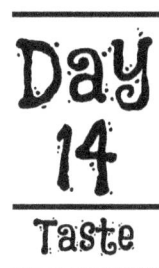

REFRESHING FIBER & PROTEIN SMOOTHIE
(Serves 2)

Ingredients:

1 cup cold coconut milk *(use a brand that is unsweetened)*
½ cup cold coconut water
½ cup cold purified water
6 frozen strawberries
4-inch piece fresh or frozen banana
2 handfuls spinach
4 tablespoons ground flax seeds *(freshly ground in a seed grinder)*
¼ cup hemp seeds
¼ cup sunflower seeds
¼ cup pumpkin seeds

Directions:

- Add all ingredients to a blender.
- Blend on high for 15-20 seconds.
- Pour into 2 glasses or glass jars.
- Remember to chew each mouthful of your smoothie.
- Enjoy!

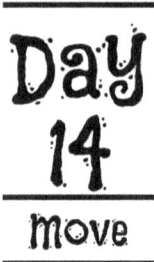

WALK UP THE STAIRS…

and then back down…

instead of taking the elevator.

(If you don't live or work near any steps or stairs, can you find some, and take a daily "hike"?)

For the next week, climb one flight of stairs (usually that's about 8 or 9 steps) each day, and walk back down.

During the following week, complete two flights.

If you live or work above the second floor of an apartment or office building, aim to walk at least half-way up and half-way down each day.

Feel the energy run through your whole body.

Your heart will become more robust, and you'll strengthen your legs.

Enjoy the fact that if the electricity ever goes out in your home or place of work, you'll already be in shape to handle the stairs.

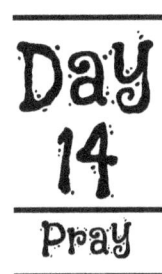

LET ME BE A GIVER

Hello God,

I admit it:

There are still times that I fall into moodiness and depression...

because instead of focusing on you and the help you can bring, I concentrate on the things that aren't working:

the test I didn't pass,

the job I didn't get,

the promotion I was passed over for,

the girlfriend who broke up with me,

the boyfriend who cheated on me,

the marriage that's falling apart,

the car that broke down,

the traffic that made me late for the meeting,

the flu,

the broken ankle,

the opportunities lost,

the weight I keep gaining and can't get rid of.

Help me to concentrate on the things that *are* working.

LET ME BE A GIVER

Give me, in the midst of any or all of these things, the ability to set aside what's bothering me --- the ability to forget about myself for a moment --- and reach out and give from what I have to someone else in need.

Help me not to hold on to my possessions with clenched fists. Help me not to stay silent when someone needs a word of encouragement. Let me live with my hands open and my mouth ready to speak encouraging words.

If I give of what I have,

my mood may be lifted,

and my circumstances may be altered.

Proverbs 11:25

*A generous person will prosper;
whoever refreshes others will be refreshed.*

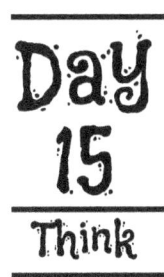

FAT: EAT IT TO LOSE IT!

Also:
EAT FAT TO STOP FEELING:
tired, sluggish, forgetful, overwhelmed, anxious, or depressed.

**What? Did you read that correctly?
Do you really need to eat fat to lose weight? And can fat really give you a better outlook on life?**

Yes! You really do need to eat fat to lose weight.
And yes, eating fat can help you feel good while you lose weight.

A research team at Washington University School of Medicine in St. Louis determined that "old" fat stored around your belly, thighs, or bottom can't be burned efficiently without "new" fat to help the process. Think of it as an example of the principle: like dissolves like. Scientifically speaking, dietary fat helps break down existing fat by activating PPAR-alpha and fat-burning pathways through the liver.

(Information about these pathways has been hidden on older "food country" travel guides. Luckily you're here with me and able to use an updated "map" for your weight-loss journey to better health and energy.)

Do you know that avoiding fats in your diet not only prevents you from burning fat in your body but can even lead to weight *gain*?

Plus, avoiding fats can be very harmful to the overall health of your organs, cell membranes, and hormones. Fat is essential for helping you absorb and process nutrients and for your body's normal growth and development.

I'm going to repeat this because I know the opposite is embedded in your brain. You've been told over and over again that you've got to stay away from saturated fat if you want to be healthy, and you've got to limit all forms of fat if you want to lose weight.

This advice is imprinted on your subconscious mind. For fifty to sixty years or more, health care professionals and the media dispensed it.

Over and over again they reinforced the idea that fats, and particularly saturated fats --- the kind you find in butter, cream, full-fat yogurt, cheese, steak, bacon, and coconut oil --- were terrible for your health --- especially if you have high cholesterol, heart disease, Alzheimer's Disease, or are overweight.

And especially if you wanted to lose weight, you were told you had to eat foods low in fat.

Meanwhile, you might have noticed something very odd.

You might have noticed that during the last fifty to sixty years, while Americans have been reducing their consumption of fats --- especially saturated fats --- diabetes, heart disease, Alzheimer's Disease, and obesity have risen sharply. People are fatter than they ever have been!

At the same time, studies conducted on populations in the Pacific Islands, Africa, and among the Inuit in Canada and Eskimos in Greenland --- societies which consume between 30% to 60% of their daily calories from fully-saturated animal fats, cream, coconut flesh, or coconut oil --- revealed that cardiovascular disease and diabetes in their populations were nearly non-existent!

Maybe you think that the Tokelauans in the South Pacific, the Massai peoples in Africa, the Inuit in Canada or the Eskimos in Greenland have nothing to do with you.

But you need to know that contemporary studies show that low-fat diets won't help you lose weight. Eleftheria Maratos-Flier, director of obesity research at Harvard's prestigious Joslin

Diabetes Center, was forced to admit that "for a large percentage of the population, perhaps 30 to 40 percent, low-fat diets are counterproductive. They have the paradoxical effect of making people gain weight."

Maybe you were one of the ones following professional advice and ate more fat-free carbohydrates to make up for the lost calories in fat. And perhaps you were one of the ones who noticed that when you did, you got hungrier, and then heavier.

Increasing evidence reveals that if you include healthy fats in your diet while removing refined sugars, processed carbohydrates, and starches from it, your food-cravings can be shut down, weight-loss can be accelerated, and you can even reverse or prevent disease.

Here's The Real Skinny on Fats:

- Your body needs fats to provide building blocks for constructing the membranes of every cell in your body. For instance, about 60% of your brain is made from fat. And about 60% of the protective wrapping (called myelin) around each of your nerves --- is made mostly from fat and cholesterol. This is one reason that current researchers now believe that those who have Multiple Sclerosis (which occurs because of damaged myelin) can benefit from eating more healthy fats.

- Your body needs fats to absorb vitamins and other plant nutrients, and to produce hormones.
  For instance, beta-carotene (which is turned into Vitamin-A in your body) needs fat (or good oils) for your body to absorb it. And you need Vitamin-A to keep your skin, mucous membranes, and eyes healthy. Lycopene, a powerful antioxidant found in watermelon, tomatoes, asparagus, and red cabbage, won't go to work fighting cancer if fat is not present.
  Should you eat your salads with no-fat dressings? NO! Oil or cheese in your salad will help your body absorb all the life-giving nutrients found in your salad's vegetables.
  (You will notice that in my green drinks I recommend

including a few nuts or seeds to provide you with a small amount of fat so that your body will absorb the vitamins in the vegetables.)

- Your body needs fats to give you the ammunition to fight against bacterial infections, viral infections, fungal infections, and other pathogens.
Conventional wisdom said that if you had any kind of open-skin wound, it was your white blood cells (like neutrophils and macrophages) that owned the entire responsibility for preventing infection.
But many failed to take into account the time it takes for white blood cells to travel to the site of the wound. Research now shows that fat stem cells under the skin are responsible for protecting against a wide range of infections until the white blood cells arrive on the scene. In fact, a fat cell can produce as many bacterial, viral and/or fungal killers as a neutrophil.

- Your body can use fats to provide you with extended energy. Think of it this way:
You use calories for energy. You get calories from the foods you eat. Carbohydrates contain 4 calories per gram, proteins contain 4 calories per gram, but fats contain 9 calories per gram. Fats are fully-loaded energy pills --- they can provide you with almost twice as much energy as can carbohydrates or protein.

Your body needs fats if you want to lose weight and keep it off. This advice is based on more than two decades of research indicating that saturated fats are actually essential to weight-loss and health. It's really not the natural fats that exist in whole foods --- foods which have been part of our human existence for centuries --- that cause weight-gain and ill health. What cause weight-gain and ill health are the "new" manufactured oils which have taken over our food supply. It's these other oils (plus an overabundance of sugar) that bear the responsibility for obesity and lousy health.

We'll talk about these other oils in two days --- when you'll be asked to take a mini-quiz --- so get ready!

The quiz will help you see for yourself how much of these very suspicious oils (or fats) that you've included in your diet cause you to gain weight and are dangerous to your health.

Where did all the bad news about fat come from?

Throughout the 20th century, research investigating the effects of consuming fats was distorted and misreported.

Two prominent scientists from the middle of the 20th century proposed theories as to why people in the United States ---- and around the world --- were gaining weight and developing heart disease. The first scientist, an American biologist and physiologist named Ancel Keys, believed the culprits of ill heart health were saturated fats; the second scientist, John Yudkin, a British physiologist and nutritionist, surmised that the culprit was sugar in the diet, and especially excessive amounts of it. As it turned out, Ancel Keys owned a dominant personality, made influential friends, and commandeered powerful political sway, three reasons why his theory became popular, drowning out every other hypothesis.

Keys' main form of "study" used a method known as epidemiology, which in his case involved either observing small groups of people and noting what they ate or collecting results from surveys that people in the studies agreed to fill out.

Normally the results from clinical trials produce more reliable results than epidemiology studies because one of the hallmarks of scientific research is to be assured that the results can be repeated. In a clinical trial, all variables can be controlled. In an epidemiological study, almost nothing can be controlled. Results from an epidemiological study can be dependent on environmental factors, time of year, and the memory and will of the subjects participating in the study. Ancel Keys became famous for his Seven Countries Study which supposedly proved a link between dietary fats, cholesterol, and heart disease. But in his investigation, Keys excluded available data that didn't comply with his pre-conceived theory. There were 22 countries in the original survey, but Keys would not include in his results countries where citizens eat a lot of saturated fat but don't die of heart disease (France, for instance), or countries where citizens eat little saturated fat but *do* die of heart disease (Israel, perhaps).

Now research shows that saturated fats (what mainline medical professionals have been misled into thinking are "the bad fats"), and even high cholesterol, are not as detrimental as once thought. Saturated fats can elevate what's been known as bad cholesterol (LDL), but studies have shown that the type of LDL that is increased is actually the large, buoyant LDL. It turns out that larger LDL particles do not appear to increase your risk of heart disease.

What might increase the risk of heart disease --- and promote the formation of fatty deposits and clogged arteries --- are the small, dense LDL particles. But small, dense LDL particles have not been shown to increase by consuming saturated fats. In fact, one large study suggested that consuming dairy products (which contain saturated fat) may actually lower your risk of cardiovascular disease. (What does increase small, dense LDL particles? A diet high in carbohydrates --- especially fructose.)

Besides having no effect on the hazardously small and dense LDL cholesterol, consuming saturated fats has been shown to elevate good cholesterol (HDL). For instance, eating a piece of steak from a free-range steer, or a portion of pure lard or bacon from a free-range pig could result in reducing your risk of heart disease.

A systematic review published in 2016 found that people over 60 years-old who have high LDL cholesterol live as long or longer than people with low LDL. The researchers who gathered this material suggested that medical professionals should re-evaluate current guidelines for preventing heart disease in older adults.

Thankfully there are now numerous books and articles available based on current research and honest reporting regarding how the fat-being-bad-myth got started.

For an historical understanding of this myth, read *Good Calories, Bad Calories* (2007), by Gary Taubes; *The Big Fat Surprise* (2014), by Nina Teicholz; *Fat for Fuel* (2017), by Joseph Mercola; and works by Sally Fallon and Mary Enig, Ph.D.

What you need to understand right now is something very, very important for your body as well as your mind.

And I'm here to give you the straight dope: the truth about fats.

Will you stay with me so new information can be planted in your brain --- new information that will replace the old, outdated, inaccurate information you've been receiving most of your life? If you do, your life will never be the same.

So here we go.

There are basically 4 types of fat that exist in our food supply: saturated fats, mono-unsaturated fats, poly-unsaturated fats, and trans-fats. All four have a *similar* chemical structure: a chain of carbon atoms, held together by single or double bonds, with one or two hydrogen atoms attached to each carbon atom.

Saturated Fats (SFs) or **Saturated Fatty Acids** (SFAs) are usually solid at room temperature and include substances like beef fat, pig fat (the truth is, lard is only about 40% saturated fat), butter, whole milk products, eggs, palm oil, and coconut oil. About 15% of the fat in an avocado is saturated fat.

Mono-Unsaturated Fats (MUFAs) are typically liquid at room temperature. Foods and oils high in MUFAs are chicken and duck fat, avocado oil (about 68% of the total fat in avocados is MUFA), nuts, peanuts, (about 50% MUFA), and olive oil.

Poly-unsaturated Fats (PUFAs) are usually liquid at room temperature and can be found in corn oil, cottonseed oil, soybean oil, safflower oil, peanut oil (about 30% PUFA on its own, peanut oil is often mixed with other oils high in poly-unsaturated fat), canola oil, flax oil, fish oil, and many nuts and seeds.

Trans-fats (TFs) come in 2 variations:

1. **Those which are created artificially in a laboratory** --- by adding hydrogen to liquid oils to make them more solid and less vulnerable to the destruction that heat, light, and oxygen cause. These types of trans-fats (also named "partially-hydrogenated oils") are solid at room temperatures and are added to many commercially

prepared foods to enhance flavor, provide a creamier texture, and extend shelf-life. (Margarine and Crisco are two examples.) *These first types of trans-fats are hugely detrimental to your health.* They increase inflammation in your body and *cause* heart disease that they were created to prevent. In fact, it is believed that many of the original studies conducted to demonstrate the "dangers" of SFs were actually performed using TFs!

2. **Those which occur naturally in meat and dairy products**. One form of trans-fat that appears naturally in meat and dairy is conjugated linoleic acid (CLA) which is now known to be quite healthy for you. *In fact, CLA can even help you become lean!*

Which fats can your body more easily use?

Because most of your body's tissues are made up of saturated and mono-unsaturated fats, your body requires more of them than poly-unsaturated fats.

This is true for all mammals.

It's also true that your body does manufacture fat from the carbohydrates and protein you eat.

But continually requiring your body to manufacture (or synthesize) large amounts of fats to build body tissue takes critical energy away from other vital processes fat is involved in performing.

Remember that you need saturated fat for:

- Breathing
- Constructing your cell membranes
- Helping your bones incorporate calcium
- Providing energy for your heart
- Protecting your liver from alcohol and other poisons
- Strengthening your immune system
- Empowering essential fatty acids to function
- Enabling your body to release toxins

So you must understand that your body absolutely needs saturated fats. Your body NEEDS the nutrients that come packaged in butter, full-fat yogurt, beef, and coconut oil.

Naturally sourced, saturated fats not only keep your heart healthy by increasing HDL levels, (which we now know is a good thing), but can also help you lose weight.

Coconut oil is an almost fully-saturated fat that can keep you satisfied and healthy, and at the same time get you to the weight you desire.

Coconut oil is known as a wonder-food because at least 50% of its fat is composed of medium-chain triglycerides (MCTs) --- also known as medium-chain fatty acids (MCFAs) --- which contain from 6 to 12 carbon atoms in their chains. Coconut oil's MCTs are considered a unique form of dietary fat because they are found in relatively few foods, yet they impart a wide range of positive health benefits.

(Short-chain triglycerides have 2 to 5 carbon atoms in their chains, and long-chain triglycerides have 14 or more carbon atoms in their chains. Both short- and long-chain triglycerides contribute significant health benefits to your body also, but are contained in other foods more abundantly than in coconut oil.)

Four of the positive benefits of MCTS are associated with helping you lose weight:

Here's how the MCTs in coconut oil help you lose weight:

1. MCTs provide about ten percent fewer calories than long-chain fatty acids (LCFAs). MCTs contain 8.3 calories per gram rather than the 9 calories per gram provided by short- or long-chain fatty acids. So when you're cooking with an MCT fat instead of an LCFA fat, you're consuming fewer calories per tablespoon.

2. MCTs provide you with quick energy without affecting your insulin levels.
After digestion, your blood will absorb MCTS through your intestines and send them straight to your liver. The liver uses MCTs for energy production and the liver's

own detoxifying processes. Unused MCTs can get sent into your muscles and other body tissues to produce energy inside of their cells. Only a small amount of MCTs converts into body fat.

3. MCTs help increase the number of calories you burn. In fact, studies suggest that MCTs can help men burn about 460 extra calories a day and women about 190 extra calories. In the process of burning fat, they promote the development of ketones.

    For many years the accepted belief has been that your brain prefers glucose (sugar) for energy. But actually, the body has two primary energy sources: glucose and/or ketone bodies. (In fact, due to the high-fat content of breast-milk, newborns are often in a state of ketosis: burning ketone bodies from the fat in breast-milk.) If you're like most people, you're probably burning glucose as a direct result of continually supplying yourself with sugar, or starches and proteins that can be turned into sugar in your body. But it is possible to shift your body away from its tendency to burn sugar toward a tendency to burn fat. You can do it by eating minimal carbohydrates, moderate proteins and…a higher amount of fats. Eating a low-carb and high-fat diet can switch your energy source from sugar to fat, or fatty acids.

    In particular, what you'd really be burning are ketone bodies: substances that result when fatty acids are broken down. Remember those tiny energy-manufacturing plants inside your cells called mitochondria that you learned about in high school? It has actually been shown that mitochondria are less efficient using glucose to make ATP (cell energy) and more efficient using ketone bodies! These ketone bodies create much less reactive oxygen and fewer destructive free radicals that can damage your cellular and mitochondrial cell membranes, proteins, and DNA.

    (Using fat for fuel has a particular benefit for your brain: burning ketones has been shown to reduce the incidences of

seizures. In fact, your brain probably contains some cells that are actually too small to hold those power-plant mitochondria. These particularly smaller cells would have to use glucose to create ATP. So a certain amount of glucose might be necessary in the diet. But in an online article, Chris Masterjohn, Ph.D., noted that in the 1980s at least two reviews were published outlining the evidence that it is possible for fatty acids to be converted to glucose when necessary.)

The benefits in knowing this for the person who wants to lose weight is that when you're burning ketones, you're safely breaking down and using up fat from the rest of your body. It does take a few weeks for your body to switch from burning carbohydrates for energy to burning fat for energy, or until you become "keto-adapted." Consuming less than 50g of carbs a day promotes ketosis, according to the Food and Agriculture Organization of the United Nations. If you are in ketosis, it means that your body is burning fat and producing ketones.

Additional compounds in coconut oil (or compounds formed when you ingest coconut oil) make it a great diet food for the following reasons:

- When you eat coconut oil containing the MCT known as lauric acid, a substance is formed called *monolaurin*. Both lauric acid and monolaurin work together to kill harmful microorganisms like bacteria, viruses and *Candida*. When you're trying to burn fat, staying healthy is significant, and coconut oil boosts your resistance to disease-causing pathogens.

- Lauric acid is the kind of fatty acid contained in breast milk --- the type of fatty acid that has been shown to make you feel satisfied when you eat it (compared to poly-unsaturated fats).

  Although lauric acid tends to raise serum cholesterol, it has a stronger impact on high-density lipoprotein (HDL) than it does on low-density lipoprotein (LDL). What happens is that lauric acid increases healthy HDL levels, and does not

substantially affect the more dangerous and compact LDL levels. Remember that high levels of HDL are beneficial for your heart health.
Lauric acid is also essential for the development and maintenance of your central nervous system, your eyes, and your brain.

- Coconut oil aids in the production and/or function of hormones. Coconut oil has a positive effect on the hormones that control your blood sugar levels and thyroid gland. For losing weight, it's essential that your hormones work properly.

- Coconut oil can help belly fat disappear. Surprising results from studies performed on both men and women show that the consumption of coconut oil is especially effective in reducing belly fat! One study, in particular, used 40 women who were fat around the middle. After 12 weeks of consuming 1 ounce (2 tablespoons) of coconut oil each day, the women enjoyed noticeable, lovely reductions in both their body-mass indexes (BMI) and the size of their waists!

The question you're probably asking now is: How much fat should you have in your diet every day (to receive all the benefits...and to lose weight)?

The American Heart Association still advocates a low-fat diet for heart health (based on faulty science and non-conclusive research) and recommends that no more than 7% of your total daily caloric intake should come from saturated fats. This means that if you're a person who eats 2,000 calories a day, you should consume per day no more than about 13.5 grams of saturated fat (a little over one tablespoon), which adds up to about 120 calories.

The Dietary Guidelines for Americans asks you to keep your *total fat intake* between 20 to 35 percent of calories, with most calories coming from sources of *poly-unsaturated and mono-unsaturated fatty acids*, such as fish, nuts, and vegetable oils.

Dr. Mercola, however, recommends that if you are insulin-resistant (and many people who are overweight and struggle to lose weight are insulin-resistant), *at least half of your diet's calories should be made up of fat*. He recommends that you obtain most fat calories from saturated and mono-unsaturated sources like coconut oil, grass-fed beef, pastured butter, pastured egg yolks, raw cacao butter, olive oil, and avocados. And he warns that only a small portion (not more than 4% of the total caloric value) should come from poly-unsaturated fats like the fat found in most nuts and seeds, and the oils that come from them. (Not all body-types can handle this amount of fat. Pay attention to your body and get a blood test done to see how a high-fat diet is affecting the inside of your body.)

After you no longer have sugar cravings, Dr. Mercola suggests that you can readjust your ratio of fats to carbohydrates, and allow for more carbs in your daily diet.

But getting one-half of your calories from saturated and mono-unsaturated fat doesn't mean that you have to eat cups of coconut oil each day.

What's a reasonable approach? The first step is to replace your other cooking fats with coconut oil. You can use coconut oil for baking as well as for sautéing and frying. Try it on your toast.

Include it in your protein drink.

Remember:
- Good Fat Burns Fat
- Good Fat Keeps You Full
- Good Fat Makes You Happy
- Good Fat Builds Muscle
- Good Fat Can Help You Maintain Your Weight

Today's Goal:

Add up to 2 tablespoons of coconut oil throughout the day: for cooking, on your toast, in your green drinks, or even in your coffee.

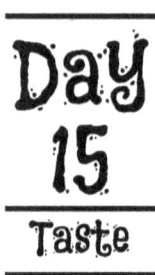

Day 15
Taste

REFRESHING FAT & PROTEIN SMOOTHIE
(Serves 2)

Ingredients:

1 cup unsweetened coconut milk
½ cup coconut water
1 cup berries *(any combination of strawberries, blueberries, raspberries, and/or blackberries)*
4-inch piece banana *(fresh or frozen)*
½ cup ice
½ cup purified water
4 tablespoons ground flax seeds *(freshly ground in a seed grinder)*
4 tablespoons cup hemp seeds
4 tablespoons cup chia seeds
2 handfuls baby kale
2 tablespoons coconut oil

Directions:

- Add all ingredients to a blender.
- Blend on high for 30 seconds.
- Pour into 2 glasses or glass jars.
- Remember to chew each mouthful of your smoothie.
- Enjoy!

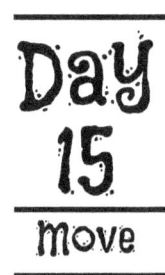

Day 15
move

TURN ON SOME MUSIC...

And dance!

When was the last time you let your body go to the feel of the beat?

Have you ever danced the waltz or the tango?

How about the twist?

What would dancing the twist look like?

Be free.

Feel the beat.

And move your body.

Make sure your dance steps include lifting yourself up onto your toes and reaching your arms out to your sides and over your head.

Dance to one whole song ---- a song you really like.

If you don't know any songs to dance to, try:

"You Make Me Feel Like Dancing" by Leo Sayer.

Or "Happy" by Pharrell Williams.

Or "Dancing Queen" by ABBA.

Or "YMCA" by Village People.

Dancing is: letting your body laugh.

Come on...you can do it!

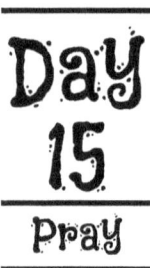

A WHOLE NEW WAY OF THINKING

Hello, God,

What an eye-opener today has been --- hearing these facts about fats.

And how contradictory the evidence is from what I expected.

I've been confused for so long as to why I've ended up gaining weight instead of losing weight while eating low-fat foods.

Understanding that foods without real fats don't easily satisfy helps me recognize one reason why I overeat...

and no wonder I've ended up still feeling hungry after ingesting whole packages of low-fat snacks...!

From this point forward, then, will you walk with me as I discover how to include in my diet what is necessary for my health?

As I include what is necessary, let me be prudent in choosing foods that aren't combined with other manufactured ingredients that can rob me of my health.

Proverbs 2: 3, 11

...indeed, if you call out for insight
and cry aloud for understanding...
Discretion will protect you,
and understanding will guard you.

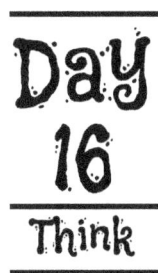

FATS to ADD:
Olive Oil & Avocado

As a review from yesterday, your body absolutely needs both saturated and unsaturated fats because of what they provide: building material for the membranes of your cells, cushion and support for your organs, help in producing the hormones your body needs, and valuable sources of energy. Fat-containing foods also help you utilize (for your overall health) crucial nutrients that can only be absorbed when fat is present. And as you learned yesterday, there are even some fats, like coconut oil, that take up the battle to fight viral and bacterial infections, too.

Yesterday we spoke about one saturated fat you can add to your diet that will help you lose weight, maintain your weight, and give you vibrant energy: raw, unrefined, coconut oil. You learned you can substitute it for other oils in all your cooking and baking recipes. You can put it on your toast and add it to your smoothie.

Today I pose to you the following question:

How many *unsaturated* fats can you add to your diet that will help you lose weight, maintain your weight, and restore your lost energy?

To answer correctly, you need to know the following information.

Unsaturated fats come in two varieties:
1. **Mono-unsaturated Fats (MUFAs):** "Mono" means "one" and these "liquidy" fats have one double bond in each chain. You find these in olive oil and avocado oil.

FATS to ADD:

2. **Poly-unsaturated Fats (PUFAs):** "Poly" means "more than one" and these fats contain two or more double bonds in each chain. This group includes the oils you know as Omega-3s and Omega-6s.

Animal fats and vegetable oils are typically made up of a mixture of saturated, mono-unsaturated, and poly-unsaturated fatty acid types.

For instance, lard (a pig fat) is about 40% saturated fat and 50% mono-unsaturated fat but does contain some poly-unsaturated fat as well. In fact, most animal fats are high in saturated fats *as well as* mono-unsaturated fats.

As you read yesterday, your body needs more saturated and mono-unsaturated fats than it does poly-unsaturated fats.

Olive oil is a mostly mono-unsaturated fat that, when added to your diet, will help you lose weight, maintain your weight, and give you vital energy.

About 72% of the fat in olive oil is a mono-unsaturated fatty acid called oleic acid (omega-9), which is believed to help reduce inflammation, and may have beneficial effects on genes linked to cancer.

Olive oil can also contain anywhere from 1.5% to 21% of poly-unsaturated fat --- which includes healthy and necessary linoleic (omega-6) and alpha-linolenic (omega-3) fatty acids.

The amount of saturated fat in olive oil can range anywhere from 7 or 8% to about 20% of its total fat content. Because of this saturated fat, olive oil is somewhat resistant to breaking down when subjected to high heat --- though what would make it more resistant would be for you to add some butter --- a fully-saturated fat --- to the pan when cooking.

*(Poly-unsaturated fats found in "vegetable" oils **are not** resistant to high heat.)*

Mono-unsaturated fats are believed to protect against heart disease, improve insulin sensitivity, help your fat cells function properly, improve your mood, strengthen your bones, reduce your risk of cancer, and help you lose weight.

Are you aware of the fact that the health of populations in the Western world is in decline --- mainly because of insulin resistance? This condition affects more than three million new people each year in the U.S. alone. A recent study showed that half of all adults in the U.S. have diabetes or pre-diabetes --- which is one result of insulin resistance. Obesity is another. (Obesity can also be the *cause* of insulin resistance.) Insulin resistance means that your body isn't able to release and process insulin in the amounts your system needs. This causes glucose to build up in your bloodstream --- leading to diabetes.

Insulin resistance and faulty fat cell function are interconnected.

You might think that a fat cell's only role is to act as a storage space for the fat produced in your body when you eat more calories than you need at the moment you eat them.

But fat cells do more. They provide heat, and they also dispense fuel when fuel is needed. The fat housed in fat cells is for times when you need extra energy because you increase your physical exertion, or because you are fasting and aren't consuming new calories to provide instant energy.

Say your body needs fuel to function, but you haven't had a recent meal. This would mean that you don't have high glucose levels in your blood...which would mean that insulin levels in your blood are low. Low insulin in your blood influences your fat cells to break down fat from your fat cells into free fatty acids and glycerol. These free fatty acids and glycerol provide fuel for the internal work of your body. (Insulin also influences fat cells to take in glucose, and fat can combine with glucose to provide energy.)

But if you are insulin resistant, your body can't tell when and how much insulin to release. Too much insulin in your bloodstream would not allow fat cells to wake up and break down their triglycerides. Too little insulin wouldn't provoke fat cells to take in glucose. The appropriate amounts of fatty acids and glycerol wouldn't be released into your bloodstream and you wouldn't get the energy or fuel your muscles, brain, and liver needed. You'd also remain...fat.

FATS to ADD:

Insulin resistance means that it's challenging to attain and maintain a healthy weight. (Please note: people with too little fat as well as people with too much fat can experience insulin resistance.)

But there is good news: you *can* increase your insulin sensitivity. And you *can* reverse fat cell dysfunction. How?

Losing weight and exercising regularly are two ways to help decrease insulin resistance. **A third way is to consume mono-unsaturated fats.** Mono-unsaturated fats can restore fat-cell function, even in the case of obesity.

Diets high in mono-unsaturated fats, particularly, have been shown to decrease a person's weight --- as well as the size of a person's waist.

Research conducted at the School of Nutrition and Health Sciences at Taipei Medical University and published in 2017 used hamsters to test the effect of using saturated, mono-unsaturated, and poly-unsaturated fats in various combinations in order to reduce weight. These studies found that for hamsters --- the most body fat was lost by those who were fed an experimental oil that was 60% mono-unsaturated.

Many studies have been conducted in countries of the Mediterranean (i.e.: Italy, Greece, and Spain) which show that **diets high in olive oil will not cause you to gain weight and can even help reduce weight**.

One study followed more than seven thousand Spanish college students over a period of two-and-one-half years, noting their olive oil consumption. A high consumption of oil was not shown to increase their weight.

One 3-year study conducted in the United States focused on subjects following a "Mediterranean Diet" (rich in olive oil) and found that the participants ended up with increased levels of antioxidants in the blood --- as well as increased weight-loss.

Yes, it's the lifestyle which comes with eating generous amounts of olive oil that promotes the ability to combat obesity, but olive oil in and of itself is a healthy fat.

Why not use extra-virgin olive oil in your salad?

Pour in a little balsamic vinaigrette or squeeze in a bit of lemon.

Add salt and pepper to taste.

Enjoy!

Attention: Olive oil overcooks at temperatures even as low as 250 degrees, which may cause oxidization, doing your body more harm than good.

So for cooking use coconut oil, butter, ghee, or lard.

Yes, lard --- the fat of pigs!

As much as 48% of the fat in lard could be mono-unsaturated. (Would you be surprised to learn that butter is about 30% mono-unsaturated? I was, too! And I bet your doctor --- as well as many magazines, newspapers and online articles --- have been telling you that butter and bacon are *harmful* because of their saturated fat *which you now know is essential for your health [see Day 15]*, and that you should eliminate them completely from your diet because they are 100% saturated, *which you now know they are not!*)

Mono-unsaturated fat --- also known as oleic acid --- or omega-9 --- is so important to include in your diet if you're trying to lose weight because oleic acid can fight against depression. (Lard, specifically, is one of the few foods that also contain high amounts of Vitamin-D, the anti-depression vitamin. The RDA for Vitamin-D is 600 IUs for the average adult, and one teaspoon of free-range lard or one slice of free-range bacon can provide as much as 500 IUs.) In health and weight-loss guides, one reason you see so many references to foods, minerals, spices, and herbs that go to work to keep your mood elevated is that guarding against depression can keep you committed to your goals when you're concerned about your weight.

Additional reasons to include mono-unsaturated fats (oleic acid or omega-9 fatty acids) in your diet involve keeping you healthy!

In 2005, a survey study conducted at Assumption University in Bangkok, Thailand reported that oleic acid has anti-cancer properties and can even decrease a person's risk of breast cancer.

FATS to ADD:

Plus, mono-unsaturated fats can protect your heart by preserving the HDL ("good") levels and lowering LDL ("bad") levels.

Besides olive oil and lard, a third mono-unsaturated fat you can add to your diet that will help you lose weight, maintain your weight, and restore your energy is the fat found in avocados.

Approximately 15% of each avocado is made up of fat (73% is water, 9% is carbohydrate/fiber, 2% is protein, and the remainder includes health-promoting vitamins and minerals). One cup of chopped avocado contains about 22 grams of fat, which equals about 198 calories.

Remember that if you are following Dr. Mercola's advice and are eating 50% of your calories as fat, and if you are consuming 2,000 calories a day, then approximately 1,000 of those calories should be from saturated or mono-unsaturated fats. One hundred ninety-eight calories from one cup of chopped avocado would leave you with 802 more calories to fill up with fat. Of all the fat in an avocado, about 73% of it is mono-unsaturated, about 10% is poly-unsaturated, and about 13% is saturated.

People who have been fed one avocado a day in test studies have been shown to have the best HDL to LDL fat blood levels.

Most researchers agree that the high levels of mono-unsaturated fat in avocado --- especially oleic acid --- play a role in these heart-related benefits. This high level of mono-unsaturated fat is similar to the amount in olive oil. But the avocado offers something more unique: something called *phytosterols*, a particular type of fat that works to reduce inflammation in your body and heart systems.

Okay, okay. What you really want to know is: can avocados help you lose weight? And the answer is: Yes!

Twenty four separate studies say yes. Not only can you reduce your body weight, but you'll also reduce your risk of factors associated with cardiovascular disease and metabolic syndrome (and weight gain promotes metabolic syndrome).

A meta-analysis of the 24 studies mentioned above evaluating diets high in mono-unsaturated fats indicated a significant reduction in triglycerides, a substantial reduction of systolic blood pressure in patients with Type 2 Diabetes, and…a considerable reduction in body weight. Additionally, there was also a significant increase in HDL (the good cholesterol). One study specifically showed the additional power dietary mono-unsaturated fatty acids have in reducing risk factors associated with cardiovascular disease and metabolic syndrome.

Other surprising foods that are rich in mono-unsaturated fats and proven to help you with weight-loss are (I'm serious): nuts and seeds!

You probably never expected nuts to be included in a weight-loss guide.

In fact, every other diet plan you've followed up to this point probably had you cutting out nuts because of their fat content. Right?

But when you cut down on fats, you probably replaced those fat calories with carbohydrates…and lost energy. For instance, maybe you stopped eating eggs and buttered toast for breakfast and substituted this higher-fat meal with a low-fat cereal?

What was the sad result of increasing your carb consumption while decreasing your fat consumption?

You probably gained more weight! (Or perhaps you lost some weight at first, but then you gained back what you lost.) Incredibly frustrating, right? So why add nuts? Aren't they *too* high in fats, which are high in calories? And haven't you always been told that if you're trying to lose weight, extra (unused) calories are what add weight? Nuts are included in my Think, Taste, Move & Pray Guide for the very reason you have probably been trying to avoid them: their fat content (plus vitamins, minerals, and phytochemicals).

Remember: consuming fat is essential if you want to lose weight and keep it off.

Adding *good* fats to your diet helps your body burn away fat from your whole body. And raw nuts can actually help prevent you from overeating.

FATS to ADD:

Raw nuts contain a "mix of omega-3 fatty acids, protein, and fiber [that] will help you feel full and suppress your appetite," says Judy Caplan, RD, a spokesperson for the Academy of Nutrition and Dietetics. The two nuts below are high in mono-unsaturated fats and are healthy additions to your weight-loss and energy-gain plan:

High-Mono-unsaturated Fat/Low-Protein Nuts:

Macadamia Nuts: have about the same level of mono-unsaturated fat (oleic acid) as olive oil, so you'll experience the same benefits of consuming olive oil that we talked about earlier today. Raw macadamia nuts also contain high amounts of Vitamin-B1, magnesium, and manganese.

Pecans: contain almost as much fat as macadamia nuts, plus an array of vitamins and minerals that fight inflammation (magnesium is one such mineral) and will boost your immune system (manganese is one such mineral).

Approximate Amount of Nuts, Protein, Calories, & Number of Grams of Mono-unsaturated Fat in One Ounce (about a handful):

Macadamia nuts: 11 nuts, 2 grams of protein, 200 calories, 17 grams of mono-unsaturated fat

Pecans: 19 nut halves, 3 grams of protein, 200 calories, 12 grams of mono-unsaturated fat

*The five nuts below are high in mono-unsaturated fats, but because of their **high-protein content**, it's helpful to limit how many of them you eat each day. (We'll discuss the reason why it's beneficial to limit the amount of protein you eat each day on Days 19 and 20.)*

High-Mono-unsaturated Fat/High-Protein Nuts:

- *Almonds*
- *Hazelnuts*
- *Cashews*
- *Pistachios*
- *Brazil nuts* (These contain almost as much poly-unsaturated fat as mono-unsaturated fat --- so it's important to limit how many Brazil nuts you eat during a day not only

because of their protein content but also because of their high percentage of poly-unsaturated fat, which we'll discuss tomorrow.)

- *Peanuts* (Peanuts are officially members of the legume family --- like beans and peas --- but since most people consider them nuts, we'll talk about them here: Peanuts can be eaten in moderation, but many problems come with them: they contain proteins that many people are allergic to, and they are often stored for long periods, allowing for mold to form on their shells --- mold which some people are allergic to, also. 60% of peanut fat is mono-unsaturated, but 30% is poly-unsaturated, and within that poly-unsaturated portion there are very few omega-3 fatty acids. We'll talk more tomorrow about why this can have a negative impact on your health.)

Approximate Amount of Nuts, Protein, Calories, & Number of Grams of Mono-unsaturated Fat in One Ounce (about a handful):

Almonds: 23 nuts, 6 grams of protein, 160 calories, 9 grams of mono-unsaturated fat

Hazelnuts: 21 nuts, 4 grams of protein, 180 calories, 13 grams of mono-unsaturated fat

Cashews: 18 nuts, 4 grams of protein, 160 calories, 8 grams of mono-unsaturated fat

Pistachios: 49 nuts, 4 grams of protein, 160 calories, 7 grams of mono-unsaturated fat

Brazil Nuts: 6 nuts, 4 grams of protein, 190 calories, 7 grams of mono-unsaturated fat

Peanuts: 28 unshelled, 7 grams of protein, 170 calories, 7 grams of mono-unsaturated fat.

How to choose nuts:

Make sure they're organically grown ---
But if you can't find organic nuts, at least select raw nuts, because roasting can damage their little nutrient-packed bodies

FATS to ADD:

--- and roasting will especially damage their beneficial omega-fatty acids.

How to prepare nuts:

The best way to prepare nuts for eating is to shell and then soak them for about 12 hours. Soaking releases their phytic acid and enzyme inhibitors, and nuts without phytic acid and enzyme inhibitors are much easier to digest.

How and when to eat nuts:

Eat a few nuts at a time.

One serving is a handful that equals about an ounce of whole nuts (or two tablespoons of nut butter made without added sweeteners, or one cup of nut milk produced without sweeteners).

Have one serving a day, before your dinner meal. Studies show that there isn't an increased benefit in eating more than that.

Going Deeper:

Canola oil --- here, there, and everywhere!

You might have heard that canola oil is high in mono-unsaturated fat. And so it is. In fact, 61% of the fat in canola oil is mono-unsaturated. But 32% is poly-unsaturated fat (and at least 21% of this is linoleic acid --- or omega-6), posing the question: is canola oil as heart-healthy as it's promoted to be?

Dr. Cate Shanahan, a physician and nutritionist who consults for the LA Lakers, advises clients to avoid canola oil for the same reasons they should avoid other "vegetable" oils.

"It's bad for you because it's a fragile, heat-sensitive oil that has been subjected to too much heat and pressure and other chemicals," says Shanahan. "It contains a high proportion of unsaturated fatty acids that undergo internal molecular reaction at high temperatures, particularly in combination with iron and oxygen, like in a frying pan, or when cooking pre-made foods in a factory, like spaghetti sauce. You end up with molecules the body simply can't deal with."

Canola oil (developed in Canada) is from a modified rapeseed plant --- part of the mustard family of plants. In the United States, canola oil was first used as an engine lubricant during World War II. Today it is used as a fuel and a base for synthetic rubber, soaps, and paints. (In actuality, many oils in our food supply are also used for these very things.) But canola oil's use as a food is a particular story.

Original rapeseed oil was extremely toxic to humans because it contained significant amounts of a poisonous substance called erucic acid. So producers developed a modified plant which now contains only trace amounts of erucic acid. The product extracted from the plant --- canola oil --- is rich in oleic acid (the omega-9 mono-unsaturated fat), low in saturated fats, and possesses a good ratio of omega-6 to omega-3 fatty acids. (We'll talk more tomorrow about why it's important to have many fewer poly-unsaturated omega-6s than poly-unsaturated omega-3s in your diet.)

Because of these qualities, producers claim canola oil is an exceptional choice for preventing heart disease.

But what producers and sellers of canola oil will not tell you is this: Studies performed in the Netherlands in 1978 were conducted to see if the new, modified canola oil would produce heart lesions in test animals --- because in previous studies using unmodified (highly toxic erucic-acid-containing) rapeseed oil, heart lesions appeared, the growth of the animals was slowed, and various organs were damaged. Experimenters combined the "new" rapeseed oil with flax oil and compared the effect against feeding them olive oil, then sunflower oil. Results were mixed. Rats genetically selected to be prone to heart lesions (meaning their heart tissue could scar easily if the muscles were damaged) developed more lesions when fed the "new" oil mixed with flax oil than those fed olive oil or sunflower oil. But for rats genetically selected to be resistant to heart lesions, there was no significant difference no matter which of the four oils they were fed.

In 1979, four neutral laboratories submitted rat experiment results to researchers at the Canadian Institute for Food Science and Technology. All four laboratories had studied the effect of the "new" canola oil as well as other oils to see how frequently heart

FATS to ADD:

lesions could be produced. What they found was this: *that high levels of omega-3 fatty acids (found in flaxseed and fatty fish) lowered the occurrence of lesions in the eyes, and saturated fats (such as palmitic and stearic acids found in beef and butter) shielded the rats against lesions in the heart!*

In 1982, the same researchers discovered something surprising when they experimented with *adding cocoa butter (a saturated fat)* to the diets of rats consuming canola oil and soybean oil. The rats in both groups had improved growth, and their heart lesions were much fewer. *The researchers concluded that a balance of fatty acids in the diet was necessary for preventing heart lesions.*

A 1995 Wall Street Journal article reported that the use of rapeseed oil (canola oil) in cooking was associated with highly increased rates of lung cancer in the women breathing the fumes. In quoting that article on their WestonPrice.org website, Mary Enig, Ph.D. and Sally Fallon explain that if the women were cooking with canola oil, eating canola oil, and breathing in canola oil fumes while eliminating saturated fats from their diets, then, of course, they might have more lung cancer. "A lack of saturates in the diet may explain the association, because the lungs can't work without adequate saturated fats."

In 1997, the Canadian researchers were back, feeding piglets with a milk replacement containing canola oil plus Vitamin-E. What did they find? Even though fed adequate amounts of Vitamin-E, the piglets showed a deficiency of Vitamin-E, a decreased number of blood platelets, larger blood platelets than normal, and longer bleeding times. (Vitamin-E is necessary for a healthy heart and for protecting cells from free-radical damage. Blood platelets aid in blood clotting and a low amount of them is a sign of anemia, and larger-than-normal platelets prevent proper blood-clotting.)

But guess what helped diminish all of these symptoms? Adding saturated fatty acids from either cocoa butter or coconut oil to the piglets' diet! These results were confirmed in another study a year later. A few years later still, researchers at the Health Research and Toxicology Research Divisions in Ottawa, Canada, fed canola oil to rats with high blood pressure. If canola oil was the only source of fat those rats were fed, then they had shortened-life-spans. Scientists surmised that what contributed to the shortened life-span of the animals were the sterol compounds in the oil, which "make the cell membrane more rigid." (A rigid membrane prevents nutrients from easily passing through.)

One main reason that the FDA once forbade the use of canola oil in infant formula is because of its inclination to hinder growth. In 2013, the multinational company, Danone, applied to the FDA to use canola oil as a source of fat in infant formula sold in the U.S. No additional evidence contrary to the results shown before 2013 were presented, yet the FDA approved Danone's request and now regards canola oil as GRAS (generally regarded as safe) for use in infant formula.

Many studies have now revealed that even though erucic acid has been bred out of the rapeseed plant, canola oil is problematic precisely *because* it contains such a high level of omega-3 fatty acids and low levels of saturated fats. Remember that you need minimal amounts of omega-3 and omega-6 fatty acids (polyunsaturated fatty acids); plus, the omega-3s in canola oil are a plant version, which your body has a tough time converting to a usable form. (See more about this on Day 17.)

When saturated fats are added to the diet of animals consuming canola oil, the detrimental effects of canola oil are lessened; but why include this oil in the first place?

Today's Goal:

Enjoy a handful of nuts, and add one half of an avocado to your salad.

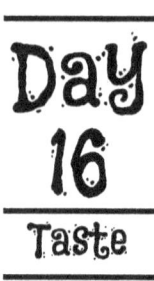

Day 16
Taste

BEFORE DINNER SNACK
(Serves 1)

Directions:

About one to one-and-a-half hours before dinner:
- Drop half of a handful of macadamia nuts (9 or 10) or pecan halves (9 or 10) plus half a handful of pistachios into a cup.
- Fix yourself a glass of chilled sparkling water with a splash of lime.
- Sit down while you partake of a pre-dinner snack.
- Remember to chew slowly.
- Enjoy!

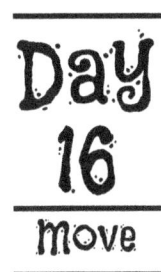

TURN ON SOME MUSIC...

And sing!

When was the last time you heard the sound of your own voice making a melody?

Do you only sing in church or at concerts?

Or in the shower?

When was the last time you sang out loud without worrying what you sounded like?

Here's how to start.

Plant your feet on the floor, a little wider than hip-width apart.

Breathe in, then, when breathing out, exhale with a great big "Ahhhhh!"

Do it again.

When you breathe in, fill up your chest.

When you breathe out with an "Ahhhh," empty your chest completely.

Now turn on a favorite song on any of your radio or digital devices, and sing out --- with feeling!

If you don't have a favorite song, try:

"Total Eclipse of the Heart," by Bonnie Tyler.

Or:

"Sweet Caroline" by Neil Diamond.

Or:
"I Will Survive" by Gloria Gaynor.
Or:
"Uptown Girl" by Billy Joel.
Or:
"You Raise Me Up" by Josh Groban.
Or:
"Praise to the Lord, the Almighty" by Fernando Ortega.
Or:
"Be Thou My Vision" by Dallán Forgall.

Singing is letting your heart laugh.
Come on.
How about a smile?

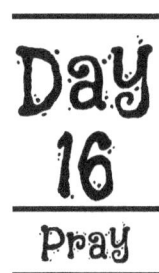

Day 16
Pray

WANTING TO HAVE A MIND OF MY OWN

Hello God,

Help me recognize that lots of people influence the way I eat.

My family, the people I work with, play with, go to church with, volunteer with --- all the people I hang out with --- and perhaps most persuasively, advertisers --- have a strong impact on me.

What these have decided I should eat is often what I end up eating. Why do I have to go along with "the crowd?"

Will you separate me from "the crowd" long enough so that I have a chance to break the chains of the foods that control me?

Help me to see that --- besides the added sugars, HFCS, refined flours, and artificial ingredients --- fast foods and packaged foods can also have lots of unhealthy fats in them. Help me to recognize that fast foods and packaged foods may not be the best foods for my weight, my energy, or my health.

Give me the strength to choose wisely.

Proverbs 13:20

Walk with the wise and become wise,
for a companion of fools suffers harm.

Proverbs 12: 26
*The righteous choose their friends carefully,
but the way of the wicked leads them astray.*

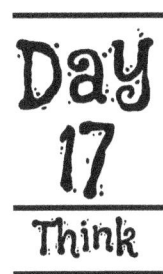

FATS TO SUBTRACT

You probably didn't think there'd be math in a guide through food country, did you?

But today's math is easy.

It's a simple subtraction question:

What other common unsaturated fatty acids (besides canola oil) should you remove from your diet to lose weight, maintain your desired weight, and give you good energy while increasing your health?

Answer: The following "vegetable" oils that are sadly advertised as healthy oils:

- soybean oil
- corn oil
- cottonseed oil
- safflower oil
- sunflower oil
- all-vegetable oil
- imitation-butter spreads (even the ones that say "trans-fat-free")

Why would I be suggesting that you subtract from your diet popular sources of poly-unsaturated fats (PUFAs) which doctors and advertisers claim can be substituted for saturated fats in equal amounts in your diet? Am I leading you astray if I insist that using them --- and especially using them in great abundance --- is dangerous to your health and counterproductive to your weight-loss goals? Will you be causing yourself harm?

Poly-unsaturated oils are harmful to you if you eat them from suspicious sources or in more than minimal quantities for three reasons:

1. They contain an unbalanced ratio of omega-6 to omega-3 fatty acids.
2. They oxidize readily, and oxidation creates free radicals in your body.
3. The processes used to produce the oils actually promote the creation of trans-fats --- whether the oils are partially-hydrogenated or not.

So I only ask that you look at the research.

As you read on Day 15, the widespread notion that saturated fats are bad for you gained prominence because of the assertive personality and influence of Ancel Keys. What Keys did not understand at the time was that cholesterol is good --- your body needs it! --- and saturated fat increases only protective HDL and non-harmful LDL. Ancel Keys questioned the impact diet could have on health right at the time refined sugar, "vegetable" oils, and products like Crisco were becoming popular in American households.

As a result of Ancel Keys' papers and presentations, doctors and other medical professionals began to proclaim that saturated fats were bad for the heart. They told their patients to stop eating butter, lard, ghee (butterfat with the water and milk solids removed), tallow (fat from cows and/or sheep), palm oil, and coconut oil.

But what could their patients replace all those fat calories with?

Ancel Keys had no problem recommending olive oil, which he observed was a main ingredient in the Mediterranean diets of populations with low cholesterol levels that he studied. Olive oil was shown to have a "better" effect than saturated fats on cholesterol levels and other blood factors. (While this is true, scientists now recognize that total cholesterol is not a marker for heart disease; it is instead the kind and number of low-density lipoproteins [LDLs] as well as the number of high-density lipoproteins [HDLs] which are better indicators.) But the problem with extra-virgin olive oil was that there weren't enough sources to meet the needs of all the people who began to clamor for it. (Furthermore, mono-unsaturated fats don't fill all of the needs of the human body.)

So scientists and profiteers searched for or developed cheaper unsaturated oils and margarines.

From the late 1950s on, then, consumption of "vegetable" oils began to skyrocket. Soybean oil, sunflower oil, corn oil, cottonseed oil, safflower oil, and even canola oil increased in availability and popularity.

Availability and popularity, however, don't mean that these oils had been (or have been) proven to be healthy for you, or shown to help you lose weight, maintain your weight, or increase your energy. The facts that most of these cooking oils were (and are) processed using heat, chemical solvents (like hexane), bleach, and deodorizers before they end up on the grocery shelf just aren't things advertisers want you to know.

And right now you, my friend, should recognize that all of these oils are very unnatural, dangerous when consumed in large amounts, and counterproductive when you are trying to lose weight. Furthermore, even when not consumed in large quantities, many studies have demonstrated that these oils can cause serious harm to your body.

Yes, your body absolutely needs PUFAs. (One type in particular builds cushioning for your nerves, makes your brain smarter, and helps to keep your body leaner.)

You probably know two PUFAs by their famous names: *omega-3 fatty acids* and *omega-6 fatty acids*. They have received a lot of attention among doctors and nutritionists, but what doesn't get a lot of attention is the fact that you only need them in relatively small quantities, and especially in the proper ratio.

Your body can actually make most of the types of fats it needs from other fats or materials within your body. But you can't manufacture omega-3 fatty acids (also called omega-3 fats or n-3 fats) or omega-6 fatty acids (also called omega-6 fats or n-6 fats). These are labeled *essential* fats --- simply because your body can't make them. Your body absolutely requires these two nutrients for the development of your brain, the proper functioning of your immune system, and the accurate regulation of your blood pressure.

If you can't make them --- even though your body, and especially your brain --- absolutely need them, where do you get these omega-3 and omega-6 fats?

The American Heart Association and the National Institutes of Health both recommend you get them from the oils that were mentioned earlier today and here: **soybean oil, corn oil, cottonseed oil, sunflower oil, safflower oil, and canola oil,** which you can purchase in various forms.

But what they're not telling you is what is becoming increasingly clear about poly-unsaturated oils --- particularly corn oil and soybean oil: they cause numerous health problems, including and especially cancer.

For instance, an animal study published in 2015 showed the effects of what a diet high in soybean oil (a poly-unsaturated fat) would produce, compared to diets high in coconut oil (a saturated fat), as well as a diet high in fructose.

Can you guess which diets had the most weight gain?

The mice fed large amounts of soybean oil! Not only that, their health became compromised by diabetes and insulin resistance. Plus, the soybean oil diet increased inflammation, obesity-related genes, and a bent toward cancer in the mice.

On the other hand, the mice fed MCT fatty acids from coconut oil, as well as mice fed peanut oil, olive oil or tea oil, reduced their body weight. Even obese mice fed a coconut oil diet had noticeably healthier blood. And neither olive oil nor MCTs from coconut oil caused significantly fatty livers.

What has been the result for people following Ancel Keys' recommendation to decrease the amount of saturated fat they're consuming? They're compensating by increasing the amount of poly-unsaturated fat in their diets. And by increasing poly-unsaturated fat, what they're really doing is increasing the omega-6 to omega-3 fat ratio of fatty acids in their diets. The ratio should be 1:1, and never more than 3:1, but in western diets, it can be as high as 20:1 or 30:1! (Tests on corn oil have found that it can be as high as 49:1!) This unhealthy ratio has been linked to heart disease, the very illness that the American Heart Association wanted (and still wants) to target, as well as cancer, inflammatory diseases, and weight gain.

Omega-6 (the prevalent poly-unsaturated fat in vegetable oils) is an essential fatty acid that is pro-inflammatory in nature, and this is a good thing when your body needs to heal its cuts, wounds, and infections.

Inflammation is part of the body's immediate response to infection or injury, but uncontrolled inflammation damages tissues. In excessive amounts, omega-6 will cause your body to stay in an inflammatory state --- and as you saw at the beginning of your journey with me, chronic inflammation is a known risk for the majority of illnesses --- including obesity.

While omega-6 is *pro*-inflammatory in nature, omega-3 is *anti*-inflammatory in nature.

As it happens, there are only so many places in any one of your cells that can hold omega fatty acids. Omega-6s compete with omega-3s to find a place to lock on to.

If there's an overabundance of omega-6s, then they're likely to fill all the places.

Why are too many omega-6s harmful?

As you just saw above, with too many 6s, there aren't enough 3s to fight inflammation.

There's an increased risk of death from heart disease, while arthritis, diabetes, and inflammatory bowel disease prosper.

Plus, when omega-3s are crowded out of your diet, you forfeit one enormous benefit if you want to lose weight: omega-3s are beneficial for weight-loss because they aid in the breakdown of fat and simultaneously reduce additional fat storage in your body. So omega-3 fatty acids shouldn't be interfered with if you want to lose weight.

Three additional surprising effects result from consuming "vegetable" oils: wrinkles, clogged arteries, and...depression.

One study by a plastic surgeon found that women who consumed mostly vegetable oils had far more wrinkles than those who used traditional animal fats. Another study found that when omega-6 oils are much more abundant in your blood than omega-3 oils, there is a high risk of severe depression. And when you want to lose weight, you've got to have the right mindset.

What about grapeseed oil?

Perhaps you've heard grapeseed oil advertised as a healthy fat because of its content of "abundant" nutrients. The reality is that it's the *seed* of the grape which contains high amounts of nutrients and antioxidants. Grapeseed oil, however, has most of those substances chemically altered or filtered out of them. The only nutrient left after the oil's intense chemical extraction process is Vitamin E, and there are much better --- more abundant and healthier --- sources of Vitamin E than grapeseed oil. (Nuts and spinach are two such foods, and they include other beneficial nutrients as well.)

As we've seen with canola oil, marketers claim that grapeseed oil is better for you because it's low in cholesterol and doesn't contain any "dangerous" saturated fats. But you already know that contemporary science has shown that saturated fat doesn't clog arteries or cause heart disease.

The big selling point for grapeseed oil is that it's high in poly-unsaturated fat.

But what manufacturers neglect to point out is that grapeseed oil is 70-75% poly-unsaturated fat, and most of that contains omega-6 fatty acids! Remember that you need to balance the ratio of omega-6 fatty acids with omega-3 fatty acids you consume, keeping the ratio as close to 1 to 1 as you can, and not greater than

3 to 1. In other words, for every three portions of omega-6, you need to eat at least one portion of omega-3. An overabundance of omega-6s in cell membranes has been shown to not only be associated with heart disease, but also with decreased cognitive function. Could there be a correlation between the current rise in Alzheimer's Disease with the increased consumption of soybean oil, corn oil, safflower oil, sunflower oil, canola oil, and grapeseed oil? I think so. A high presence of omega-6 fatty acids also increases inflammation, which in itself is associated with many more diseases --- including obesity!

So what's left for the advertisers to advertise? That this oil has a "high smoke point," making it a "healthy" cooking oil. (Smoke point, by the way, is the temperature at which the the fat produces a thin, continuous stream of bluish smoke under controlled conditions. Until a smoke point is reached, fats supposedly remain stable (or safe). But once passing the smoke point, components can break apart, free radicals reacting to oxygen released, and compounds formed that can harm your cells and even your DNA, according to the Health Science Academy. These polar compounds have been linked to Alzheimer's and Parkinson's Disease.) A smoke point can vary greatly depending on the volume of oil being heated, the size of the container, and the amount of "free" acids or extraneous compounds in the oil. Industrial processing removes a lot of the free acids and extraneous compounds, creating a higher smoke point. So some oils can break down and are dangerous to consume even before the smoke point is reached.

Poly-unsaturated fats are precisely the kind of fats that are unstable when heated and prone to oxidize (break down) easily. The smoke point doesn't tell you how stable an oil is. The amount of poly-unsaturated fatty acids it contains as well as the amount of processing the oil has undergone determine the stability of an oil. Some oils are so high in poly-unsaturated fatty acids that merely being exposed to light and oxygen can cause them to break down. Others break down by being heated over and over again. When poly-unsaturated oils break down, they become rancid, and eating rancid oils provides your body with lots of extra free radicals which --- besides being able to make you sick

--- can wreak serious havoc in your cells. (The dangers include the destruction of cell membranes, interruption of cell function, and even cell mutation that can lead to cancer).

The *Unnatural* Saturated Fat in Our Food Supply:
Man-Made Trans-Fat
(Worse Than An Over-Abundance of Poly-Unsaturated Fat)

If omega-3 fatty acids are successful in aiding weight-loss, you should be aware of hazardous yet very abundant *anti*-omega-3 fatty acid substances in your food sources that promote weight gain: trans-fats. One reason trans-fats are linked to obesity and weight gain is because they interfere with your body's use of beneficial omega-3 fatty acids. They also increase inflammation in your body, which increases your risk of diabetes.

Trans-fats are formed when poly-unsaturated oils are chemically altered to become "partially solid" --- or "partially-hydrogenated." Partially-hydrogenated fats have been used a lot commercially because they have a longer shelf-life and give flakiness to baked goods and crispness to crackers and chips. They provide more texture and less "oiliness" to most foods.

But even though partially solid, partially-hydrogenated vegetable and seed oils (otherwise known as trans-fats) may deliver a longer shelf-life to foods, they do not give *you* a longer shelf-life.

Medical and scientific communities are now fairly united in the opinion that these partially-hydrogenated vegetable and seed oils --- or trans-fats --- should be avoided. This includes margarine and "vegetable spreads," the type of food that for almost half a century was touted as THE diet food everyone was supposed to use to maintain a healthy weight. And this also includes partially-hydrogenated oils in processed foods. In November 2013, the U.S. Food and Drug Administration (FDA) finally, and bravely, advertised that partially-hydrogenated oils are no longer "Generally Recognized as Safe" in human food. Food companies were required to remove all partially-hydrogenated oils from their products by mid-2018. But beware: a Nutrition Facts label can state that it has "0 grams of trans-fat" even if the food product contains up to 0.49 grams of trans-fat per serving. (And the serving size can be unreasonably small; one person would normally consume two or three times as much.) This means that even if the label says "zero grams of trans-fat," a product still might contain small amounts of trans-fat if it is created using hydrogenated oils.

Going Deeper:

Is Crisco your go-to fat/oil for cooking or baking?

Then, my dear friend, please understand the following:

Proctor & Gamble began producing Crisco in 1911 and advertised it as a newer and cheaper (cheaper than lard or coconut) industrial fat. Crisco was praised for the flaky texture it gave to baked goods and its ability to accept high temperatures for frying. Crisco was first made by extracting oil from the seeds of cotton and then partially hydrogenating that liquid oil into a solid.

P&G employed a very influential advertising company to extol the benefits of this "clean" and inexpensive "vegetable" oil.

But what P&G didn't tell anyone at the time was that cottonseed oil is at least 50% omega-6 fatty acids. Later P&G substituted cottonseed oil with soybean oil. But Crisco's manufacturing processes for both types, unfortunately, resulted in a product containing a high amount of "trans-fats" --- which the FDA now warns you to avoid.

Once again in 2017, Crisco changed its recipe to provide for fewer trans-fats. If you examine the ingredients on a new can of this "all-vegetable" shortening, however, you'll see that it contains soybean oil, fully-hydrogenated palm oil, partially-hydrogenated palm and soybean oils, and stabilizers. Because of the use of the partially-hydrogenated oils, trans-fats will be present in Crisco, even though the ingredient list shows that in one serving of Crisco shortening there are zero grams of trans-fats. This is because of what I wrote above: a Nutrition Facts label can legally state that it has "zero grams of trans-fat" even if the food product contains up to 0.49 grams of trans-fat per serving. So if you eat any more than one serving (1 tablespoon) of Crisco, you might be consuming more than 0.5 grams of trans-fats. From a typical recipe, one cookie contains about one tablespoon of shortening. Eating two cookies would take you into the danger zone.

FATS TO SUBTRACT

Are trans-fats hiding in your food supply?

Today's Goal (Part-A):

Reading may be the most important step you take in *Becoming Lean and Free*. **Read the ingredient labels on all food packages you have in your cupboards.** The last time you investigated packaged-food labels, you were on the lookout for all the ways sugar could hide in the foods you eat. Today, **search for oils and all their relatives**.

Be on the lookout for: "shortening," "hydrogenated" or "partially-hydrogenated oil" --- all ways trans-fats can hide in the foods you eat. The higher up on the list these ingredients appear on the packaging, the more trans-fat the item contains.

Here's a cheat sheet to help you recognize foods that might have lost their labels but would probably contain a manufactured form of trans-fat known as partially-hydrogenated oil:

- Baked goods: most cakes, cookies, pie crusts, and crackers contain shortening, which is usually made from partially-hydrogenated vegetable oil.
- Ready-made frosting
- Snacks: potato, corn and tortilla chips often contain trans-fat. And while popcorn can be a healthy snack, many types of packaged or microwave popcorn use trans-fat to help cook or flavor the popcorn.
- Fried food: foods that require deep frying --- French fries, doughnuts, fried chicken --- can contain trans-fat from the oil used in the cooking process. (Many fast-food restaurants --- and even many slow-food restaurants! --- often use trans-fats to deep fry their foods because the oils can be used over and over again.)
- Refrigerator dough: products such as canned biscuits and cinnamon rolls often contain trans-fat, as do frozen pizza crusts.
- Creamer and margarine: non-dairy coffee creamers and stick margarines also may contain partially-hydrogenated vegetable oils.

Besides eliminating trans-fats from your diet with the help of new government regulations, I'd like to know if you're willing to go for extra-credit?

Are you willing to choose to stop using unhealthy and counter-productive "vegetable" oils on your own? If so, act on:

Today's Goal (Part-B - if you are brave):

Will you check and remove from your refrigerator and cupboards all the products containing the following oils?

- Soybean Oil
- Corn oil
- Cottonseed Oil
- Safflower Oil
- Sunflower Oil
- All-Vegetable Oil
- Imitation Butter Spreads
- Hydrogenated Oil

If you don't have the power to immediately stop using your current inventory of these products because you think you'll be "wasting" food, go back over the harm eating too many omega-6s does to your health. Imagine the time wasted in feeling sick, going to the doctor, and undergoing operations. Imagine the depression you'll be free of and the mental clarity that will return when you eliminate the high amount of damaged omega-6 fatty acids from your diet.

If and when you do muster up the power to eliminate --- or at least phase out --- the above oils (with their dangerously processed omega-6s) from your diet, you're going to find that they're in an awful lot of foods.

In fact, there are so many packaged foods that contain either added sugar or some sort of "vegetable" oil, that if you eliminated all of them from your refrigerator and cupboard both would be rather empty.

Which would be a good thing.

Because then you'd have room for "whole" foods.

Whole foods are those foods that haven't been cut up, boxed up, wrapped up, or canned-in by food-processing companies. Whole foods are things like heads of lettuce, stalks of celery, tubers of cucumbers, fresh organic carrots, fresh broccoli, green beans, onions, sweet potatoes, and squash that you cut up yourself and cook together in a pot or eat as a salad.

Are you willing to buy fresh foods from the market and prepare them yourself?

Are you willing to at least begin today by making your own salad and salad dressing?

Are you willing to buy fresh chicken or fish and broil or bake it with a little butter, garlic, paprika, salt, and pepper?

Today's Goal (Part-C):

Replace all cooking oils with saturated fats.

For cooking with heat, saturated fats such as coconut oil, butter, ghee, lard, beef tallow, or mutton tallow are the most stable.

Replace all salad oils with healthy mono-unsaturated fats.

For salads, you can use cold-pressed oils such as olive and avocado, or even sesame oil (if the label specifically states that it is cold-pressed and you keep it refrigerated).

Today's Goal (Part-D):

You're probably wondering by now about other good sources of poly-unsaturated fats. Where are healthy omega-3 and omega-6 fatty acids hiding? If "vegetable oils" are dangerous to your health and unprofitable for losing weight, where do you find safe PUFAs? And if you need them so badly, are they easy to include in your diet?

What about the amount --- how much is too much?

Based on available evidence for omega-3s, you should be aiming for 1 gram/day of combined eicosapentaenoic acid (EPA) and docosahexaenoic acid (DHA). During pregnancy and lactation at least 300mg/day are needed. (EPA and DHA are animal-sourced omega-3s, and ALA is plant-sourced omega-3 which your body converts to EPA and DHA.)

If you choose today's "before-dinner snack" from LIST 1 below, you'll be consuming nuts or seeds containing a high amount of ALA. These foods have also been shown to help you lose weight. You'll learn more about the fascinating weight-loss benefits of omega-3 fatty acids tomorrow.

LIST 1 (High in ALA Omega-3 Fatty Acids)

- *English Walnuts*: 14 halves: 2.5 grams of omega-3 fatty acids, 10.6 grams of omega-6 fatty acids, 13.4 grams of additional poly-unsaturated fat, 4.3 grams of protein, 190 calories. (The ratio of omega-3s to omega-6s in English walnuts is about 1 to 4, which is higher than your goal of keeping the ratio close to 1 to 1; but it is still lower than the 1 to 20 ratio you often see, and is allowable because it is one of the few vegetarian sources of omega-3s.)

- *Chia Seeds* (2 tablespoons, whole): 4.9 grams of omega-3 fatty acids, 1.6 grams of omega-6 fatty acids, 7.2 grams of poly-unsaturated fat, 4 grams of protein, 137 calories.

- *Flaxseeds* (2 Tablespoons, ground): 3.2 grams of omega-3 fatty acids, 0.4 grams of omega-6 fatty acids, 4 grams of other poly-unsaturated fat, 2.6 grams of protein, 74 calories.

- *Flaxseed Oil* (2 Tablespoons, cold-pressed and refrigerated): 14.9 grams of omega-3 fatty acids, 3.5 grams omega-6 fatty acids, 18.5 grams of poly-unsaturated fat, 0 grams of protein, 248 calories.

- *Hemp Seeds* (2 Tablespoons, whole): 2 grams of omega-3 fatty acids, 5 grams of omega-6 fatty acids, 6.5 grams of poly-unsaturated fat, 7 grams of protein, 114 calories. Hemp seeds also contain 0.6 grams of Super Omega-6 Gamma Linolenic Acid (GLA) and 0.3 g Super Omega-3 Stearidonic Acid (SDA).

If you choose today's "before-dinner snack" from LIST 2, you'll be consuming nuts or seeds containing a high amount of omega-6 fatty acids (which do NOT include significant amounts of EPA or DHA). These nuts and seeds have also been shown to help you lose weight (but because of their high omega-6 content, you should balance the amount you eat with foods high in omega-3s). The ratio should be one omega-3 to one omega-6. It is still safe to have a ratio of one omega-3 to three omega-6s, but try not to go higher. And remember that you *need* minimal amounts of all omega fatty acids --- only about 5 grams of oil, total.

LIST 2: (High in Omega-6 Fatty Acids)

- *Brazil Nuts* (1 oz or 6 nuts): 5.7 grams of omega-6 fatty acids, 0.05 gram of omega-3 fatty acids, 5.8 grams of other poly-unsaturated fat, 4 grams of protein, 184 calories.
- *Cashews* (17 whole pieces): 2.18 grams of omega-6 fatty acids, 0.017 gram of omega-3 fatty acids, 2.2 grams of other poly-unsaturated fat, 5 grams of protein, 160 calories.
- *Sunflower Seeds* (¼ cup): 8.07 grams of omega-6 fatty acids, 0.03 grams of omega-3 fatty acids, 8.10 grams of other poly-unsaturated fat, 7.27 grams of protein, 204 calories.
- *Pine Nuts* (¼ cup): 6.9 grams of omega-6 fatty acids, 0.22 gram of omega-3 fatty acids, 7.2 grams of other poly-unsaturated fat, 4 grams of protein, 190 calories.
- *Pumpkin Seeds* (1/4 cup): 6.7 grams of omega-6 fatty acids, 0.04 grams of omega-3 fatty acids, 6.7 grams of other poly-unsaturated fat, 7 grams of protein, 151 calories.
- *Sesame Seeds* (2 tablespoons): 6.8 grams of omega-6 fatty acids, 0.01 gram of omega-3 fatty acids, 6.9 grams of poly-unsaturated fat, 5 grams of protein, 170 calories.

Remember that any seed or nut that contains four or more grams of protein per serving-ounce is considered a "high in protein" food. Eating protein will help you lose weight; you just need to make sure you have enough, but not too much…like Goldilocks. More about this tomorrow.

Today's Overall Goal: To lose weight: eliminate detrimental fats and have at least one serving (one handful) of raw, tasty nuts.

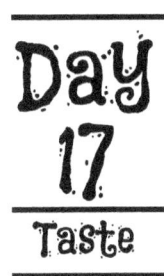

SCRUMPTIOUS LUNCH SALAD
(Serves 2)

Ingredients:

2 large handfuls mixed salad greens, chopped
¼ large yellow pepper *(washed & cut into 1/4 inch pieces)*
½ cup carrot strings
½ cup chopped cucumber
1 Haas avocado *(peeled and chopped)*
2 tablespoons sunflower seeds
1 tablespoon lemon juice
4 tablespoons extra-virgin, cold-pressed olive oil
1/2 teaspoon powdered kelp
pink Himalayan salt & pepper to taste

Directions:

- Put all ingredients into a large bowl and mix.
  You can add 6 ounces of wild Alaskan canned salmon or wild-caught Alaskan sardines to this salad for a complete meal.
- Serve with a slice of sprouted grain bread or a handful of gluten free crackers.*
- If you are able, let this meal be the first meal of the day.
- If you can wait until noon to eat it, all the better.

*Few crackers on the market today contain healthy oils. Look for ones made with coconut oil, butter, ghee, olive oil, or palm oil. Otherwise, choose brands that don't use any oil at all. Check www.kriswilliamswellness.com for healthy brands.

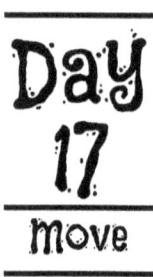

Day 17
move

USE CAN WEIGHTS...
to strengthen your arms.

Choose two 16-ounce cans of vegetables or soup and hold one can in each hand.

Stand with feet on the floor, hip-distance apart.

Lower the cans so your arms are straight on either side of your legs. Then, while holding the cans, extend both arms straight out in front of you to shoulder height. Alternate lifting/lowering the cans with palms of hands facing downward.

Do for 10 times each.

Next while holding the cans, extend arms straight out to your sides with palms of hands facing downward.

Lower and lift both arms to shoulder height 10 times.

Next, let your arms hang down on either side of your legs and turn palms of your hands to face upward while holding the cans.

Alternate bending your right arm up while squeezing the can, then bending your left arm up while squeezing the can.
Curl up each arm 10 times.

Next bend forward at the waist with your arms extended out behind you. While holding the cans, palms of hands should face inward.

Lower your forearms at the elbow, then extend back while feeling the muscles at the back of your arms tighten.

Do for 10 times.
Stand upright.
Return the cans to your pantry...

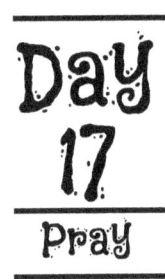

GIVE ME THE GRACE TO FORGIVE

Hello God,

Sometimes other people offend me.

They're impatient with me and insensitive to how much the harsh things they say hurt me.

They interfere in my life when I don't want them to, or when I want their attention, they ignore me.

They don't respect me or appreciate the work I do.

There are even times it's just the weird things they do or their strange idiosyncrasies that aggravate me.

I admit that there are times when I let these offenses of others fester inside me.

I feel wronged, and self-pitying or vindictive thoughts populate my brain.

Then it's hard preventing unkind and unloving words from escaping my lips.

My thoughts burn into my belly, and my words burn into the soul of the person I say them to.

I get belly-burn and give heart-burn.

God, will you forgive me for so often focusing on how I'm offended?

Will you give me the willingness to let go?

Will you help me not take offense and not be resentful when

others don't treat me as I want or expect?

Give me the grace to excuse other people's weaknesses.

Let me begin to understand that love is a verb, and real love is patient, ready to excuse, and inclines a person to speak with kindness…

because I know that even healthy food with an unkind heart won't make me healthy.

Proverbs 15:17

*Better a small serving of vegetables with love
than a fattened calf with hatred.*

I Corinthians 13:4-7

*Love is patient, love is kind.
It does not envy,
it does not boast,
it is not proud.
It does not dishonor others,
it is not self-seeking,
it is not easily angered,
it keeps no record of wrongs.
Love does not delight in evil but rejoices with the truth.
It always protects,
always trusts,
always hopes,
always perseveres.*

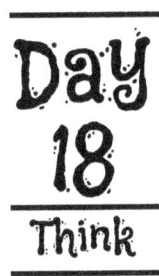

FISHING FOR THE RIGHT FOODS

Eating fat combined with protein is an effortless way to include many essential nutrients into your diet.

Eating fat combined with protein is also an effortless way to lose weight, maintain your weight, and gain energy, too.

On Day 16 we talked about olive oil, avocadoes, macadamia nuts, and pecans that are beneficial to include in your diet because of their high content of mono-unsaturated fat.

You saw that mono-unsaturated fat is an excellent fat for you to consume because most of your body's tissues are made up of mono-unsaturated fats and saturated fats, and your body requires more of them than poly-unsaturated fats. Mono-unsaturated fats will help you feel full and give you the energy you need.

You also reevaluated other common nuts --- almonds, cashews, pistachios, hazelnuts, Brazil nuts, and peanuts --- that aren't only high in mono-unsaturated fats but are also high in protein.

You were asked to limit your intake of almonds, cashews, pistachios, hazelnuts, Brazil nuts, and peanuts --- as well as milk or nut butters made from them --- because of their high-protein content. And in a short while (I promise you) we're going to talk about why.

Right now I want to do just a little more review. Will you stay with me?

Yesterday we talked about poly-unsaturated fats, the oils that contain them, and the dangers they pose to your health and weight-loss efforts. You were asked to eliminate from your diet these major offenders --- soybean oil, corn oil, canola oil, cottonseed oil, safflower oil, sunflower oil, all-vegetable oil, and imitation butter spreads --- because the high-heat and chemicals used to process them destroy their precious, but fragile, fatty acids. Remember, you need unheated, unprocessed poly-unsaturated fats in small quantities and in the right proportions to be able to absorb them without dangerous consequences.

Yesterday you learned that raw nuts and seeds are great foods to eat because they provide safe packaging for their poly-unsaturated fats. When you eat nuts and seeds raw, then you're assured their oils haven't been subjected to destructive heat or manipulated with dangerous chemicals.

You learned about *four sources of poly-unsaturated fats that are high in essential omega-3 fatty acids*: English walnuts, chia seeds, flaxseeds, and hemp seeds.

And you also learned about *five sources of poly-unsaturated fats that are high in essential omega-6 fatty acids*: Brazil nuts, sunflower seeds, pine nuts, pumpkin seeds, and sesame seeds.

In a minute I'm going to reveal to you the best foods for you to choose when you want to combine high-quality protein with essential fatty acids your body requires for health and weight-loss.

But first, you need a bit more information that scientists have discovered about omega-3 fatty acids.

Diving deeper:

The three types of omega-3s that you heard about yesterday come in long- and short-chain varieties.

- *Two long-chain omega-3 fatty acids* are known as eicosapentaenoic acid (EPA) and docosahexaenoic (DHA). EPA and DHA are the building blocks for hormones that decrease inflammation (when your body has a chronic infection), reduce the risk of blood clotting (when your blood vessels are hardening), and reduce cell proliferation (when abnormal, cancerous cells want to multiply).

- *One short-chain form of omega-3* is called alpha-linolenic acid (ALA). It's the only omega-3 found in land plants. So the four sources of omega-3 fatty acids you reviewed yesterday --- English walnuts, chia seeds, flaxseeds, and hemp seeds --- contain short-chain ALA only. They do not contain EPA or DHA.

What makes ALA distinctive is that it must be converted to the long-chain DHA and EPA by your body before it can be put to use.

And the sad part about this bit of science is that the metabolic conversion process can only convert small amounts of ALA into EPA, and even smaller amounts into DHA.

Note: Like EPA and DHA, omega-6 fatty acids are also needed to construct hormones, but --- am I emphasizing this too much? --- omega-6-type hormones mostly produce an opposite effect than what omega-3-type hormones produce. If you have the right balance of omega-6 fatty acids, you can build hormones that: increase inflammation when your body needs to fight acute infection, increase blood clotting when you have an open wound, and increase cell proliferation when you need healthy cells to grow.

Since both omega-3 and omega-6 fatty acids are needed to maintain optimum health, you must consume both, in a correct balance. *Our bodies were created to enjoy one omega-3 portion of fat with no more than three portions of omega-6 fat.* (I'm repeating these facts because repetition helps reinforce our memories...) If you have too many omega-6 fatty acids, inflammation within your body gets out of control, blood-clotting increases, blood vessels constrict, cancer cells proliferate, and that weight you want to get rid of? It stubbornly stays.

> **Four big reasons** *you need to make sure* **you get the right amount of omega-3s in your diet:**

- Omega-3s are considered the "happy" fat. They help fight anxiety and depression.
- Omega 3s can make your brain healthier and you smarter!
- Omega-3s can help raise beneficial HDL for heart health.
- Omega-3s reduce liver fat and inflammation, helping you lose weight .

What are the best sources of omega-3 fats?

The fact is, your body needs all three omega-3 fats (EPA, DHA, and ALA), and for this, you need both animal AND plant sources.

Vegans (vegetarians who eat no foods derived from animals, including eggs and milk) will argue that you can acquire all of the omega-3 fats you need from the plant sources listed above (flaxseed, hemp seeds, chia seeds, and English walnuts), but this may not be possible.

Even though your body can convert ALA into EPA and DHA — it works its conversion magic in small quantities only. You just won't be able to consume enough plant substances to meet all your body's omega-3 fat requirements. One possible solution is to take supplements from sea algae.

Scientists have learned that although microalgae contain DHA only, if you take it in supplement form, your EPA levels will also increase substantially. This is especially important for vegans.

How can you combine first-rate protein with essential fatty acids your body requires for health and weight-loss?

- Look for omega-3 ALA in English walnuts, flaxseed, hemp seeds, and chia seeds.
- Look for omega-3 EPA and DHA in fatty, cold-water fish such as salmon, mackerel, herring, sardines, krill oil, or from sea algae if you're a vegetarian.

I personally take krill oil trolled from the Antarctic. Dr. Mercola states that Antarctic krill contain a highly nutritious blend of omega-3 fats, antioxidants, and choline. The omega-3 fats found in pure krill oil are predominantly EPA and DHA, the same as what's found in cold water fish. A typical krill oil dose has less EPA and DHA than fish oil, but the omega-3 fats in krill oil are bonded to phospholipids, as opposed to what are known as triglycerides in fish oil. While triglycerides don't disperse easily in water, phospholipids do, which means that phospholipids easily blend in stomach fluids. So if you're burping up fish oils, it's probably because they're bonded to triglycerides. You'll probably digest omega-3s bonded to phospholipids more easily. (Studies also confirm that the omega-3s found in sea microalgae are in triglyceride form, the same as those found in fish oil.)

The benefit of eating fatty fish is that while you're consuming healthy and helpful omega-3 fatty acids, you're also consuming valuable protein...

which every human being needs to stay alive.

The truth is, you must have enough protein in your diet, but not too much (like Goldilocks), because too much protein can cause damage to your kidneys and has been shown to be a contributing factor in the growth of cancer cells.

Plus, you need just enough protein because your body can't store amino acids or protein as such. Your body stores extra protein as fat. So if you're trying to lose weight, you need just enough protein, but not too much.

I know you've seen body-builders include large amounts of extra protein in their diets as they strain to build bigger and stronger muscles. Body-builders continually tear down muscle and then are left with the need to consume calories from some form of food to build their muscles back up. They need extra calories and choose protein for their calorie source.

And they choose protein for a reason.

Without protein, their muscles could not grow, their tendons would not maintain flexibility, and their hormones would lose the tools they need to function.

You've probably watched those body-builders wondering if your body needs protein even if you don't have a consistently demanding exercise program. And the answer is: you do!

Even if you're not exercising at a frenetic rate or lifting a ton of weights every other day, your body should have some protein every day.

Twenty percent of your body weight is from protein, and it's found in every cell of your body --- and every cell uses it to build and maintain its structure. Without protein, your bones and muscles would not grow, you would lose flexibility, and you would not be able to produce enzymes or hormones (leaving you with wildly fluctuating moods, the inability to maintain a correct body temperature, and a lack of sexual desire).

Protein helps your body regulate the movement of fluids and minerals in and out of cells and even enables you to fight infection with the antibodies it builds.

Without protein, you wouldn't survive.

So if you're planning to lose weight by eliminating good sources of protein from your diet, don't!

Because the thing is, eating protein can even help you lose weight. The reason?

Protein helps you stay committed to your plan.

Answer this:

What's the #1 reason people quit their diets?

Food cravings!

A recent survey conducted by a food company in the UK found that food cravings cause 40% of dieters to quit within the first week, and another 40% to drop out within the first month.

What's one way to fight food cravings?

A 2011 issue of Obesity magazine featured a study conducted by researchers at Purdue University (funded by the National Pork Board, the American Egg Board, the Purdue Ingestive Behavior Research Center, the National Institutes of Health's Indiana Clinical Center, and the Translational Sciences Institute). They wanted to find out what effect a high-protein diet had on losing weight.

Their test study targeted twenty-seven obese and overweight men and divided them into high-protein and normal-protein consumption groups.

All subjects were fed 2,400 calories a day, about 750 calories less than they were used to eating.

The eating plan for the high-protein group contained 25% protein from pork and egg products, 49% carbohydrates, and 26% fat.

The normal-protein group's program provided 14% protein, 60% carbs, and 26% fat.

After 12 weeks, researchers found that the high-protein group experienced greater fullness throughout the day...even though they ate the same number of calories as the normal-protein group. The desire to eat late-night snacks was also reduced.

In a similar study conducted on women, all subjects lost about 18 pounds after 12 weeks, but the high-protein group did it comfortably and reported they were more likely to stay on the diet.

Protein goes right to work combating the thing people most hate about dieting: hunger!

A second benefit is that protein in your diet promotes good sleep at night. And good sleep typically helps weight-loss.

"Our research suggests that what you eat while losing weight can influence whether or not sleep improves," said Wayne W. Campbell, a professor of nutrition science at Purdue University. "And consuming a higher-protein diet improved sleep."

The first of two studies that Campbell and his team conducted to verify if a high protein diet could improve sleep found that the source of protein didn't matter. A person could eat vegetable or animal protein and still be able to rest equally well. What mattered was that, for a good night's repose, both vegetarian and non-vegetarian eaters had to eat an equal percentage of calories from protein.

The second study — one of the longest of its kind to look at the effect of protein intake on sleep — illustrated that ability to rack up all "forty winks" was higher for individuals on a high protein diet compared with those consuming lower amounts of protein.

Protein sources didn't matter, but the amount of protein did.

Besides settling you into a good night's slumber, if the amount of protein you include in your day adds up to about 30% of all the calories you eat, then you can boost your metabolism. Which means you'll be burning more calories while you're awake --- even up to 100 calories a day --- compared to what you would burn if you were eating a very low protein diet.

Plus, protein may be able to reduce your appetite, providing additional support to help you lose that stubborn weight you can't seem to get rid of. Because you remain satisfied for more extended periods (longer than the satisfaction time that carbohydrates bring), you end up eating fewer calories.

What about eating more often during the day? Don't authorities recommend eating five small meals during the day (rather than three larger ones) to stave off hunger and lose weight?

Get ready for the answer.

Research (conducted at Purdue University and reported in *Obesity* magazine in 2011) showed that the 5-small-meals-a-day plan doesn't work...for everyone.

As long as subjects in the trial were consuming a high-protein diet, the number of daily meals made no difference in how satisfied each member felt.

So, if you're looking to suppress your appetite and increase your fat-burning, you'll want to choose a diet with fat that includes more protein than carbohydrates.

And one more secret that I want to share with my older, more mature reading audience: Additional research found that higher-protein eaters who are 50 years old or more preserved more muscle mass than low-protein eaters while they were losing weight. Imagine! There is a way to become more lean, gain energy, and stay strong all at the same time!

Now the question is, what are good sources of protein?

We've already looked at seeds, nuts and the milk made from them --- all vegetarian sources that include some protein.

But are there other healthy, more complete, alternatives?

Yes!

Which is why we're talking about fish.

The good thing about including salmon, mackerel, herring, and sardines in your diet is that these fishes contain protein *plus* omega-3 fatty acids. An oily fish is a "full-to-the-gills" nutrition pill that will help you lose weight, maintain a good weight, and give you energy.

The best, most nutrient-rich salmon is that which is caught wild from the Pacific Ocean. Fish to avoid are any farmed in the Atlantic Ocean (including salmon). Farmed fish can be contaminated from the waters they swim in, and the feed they receive is often filled with bad/rancid oils and food waste products.

How much protein do you need?

The DRI (Dietary Reference Intake) for the average person is figured this way: eat about 0.36 grams of protein for every pound of your body weight.

For instance, if you weigh 150 pounds, then you should be eating 54 grams of protein a day.

Most people need at least 3 ounces at each meal, adding up to about 54 to 81 grams of protein per day.

But this is for maintaining your weight.

If you want to lose weight, then you should eat about 0.7 grams of protein per pound of your body weight. If you weight 140 pounds, you would need to consume about 98 grams of protein daily.

If you want to gain muscle and are exercising with weights, then you should eat 0.8 grams of protein for each pound of body weight.

And just so you know, seafood contains an average of 6 to 9 grams of protein per ounce.

Tomorrow you'll find out more options for protein, and how many grams of protein are in each ounce. Oh, the things you have to look forward to!

Today's Goal: Try a piece of baked Alaskan salmon. You'll receive a generous amount of protein and omega-3 fatty acids.

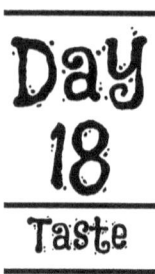

SUCCULENT SALMON DINNER
(Serves 2)

Ingredients:

2 pieces wild Alaskan Salmon *(each piece = 6 ounces)*
10 stalks asparagus
1/2 cup uncooked brown or black rice
first cold-pressed virgin olive oil
1 tablespoon butter
coconut oil
garlic powder
pink Himalayan salt & pepper to taste

Directions:

For Rice:
- Melt 1 teaspoon of coconut oil in heavy saucepan, then add rice.
- Stir rice over medium heat until slightly browned.
- Add 1 1/8 cup water & bring to boil.
- Cover & reduce heat to simmer.
- Cook for about 35-40 minutes, or until water is evaporated & rice is soft.

For Salmon:
- Coat the bottom of a glass pyrex dish with coconut oil.
- Lay salmon in dish and top with small pats of butter.
- Season with garlic powder, salt & pepper.
- Place salmon dish in a preheated 350-degree oven.
- Bake for 15 minutes, or until desired doneness.

For Asparagus:
- In the same oven as the salmon:
- Place asparagus on a cookie sheet rubbed with a bit of coconut oil.
- Roast for about 10 to 15 minutes, or until gently browned.
- When done, drizzle a bit of olive oil over the asparagus for flavor.
- Add salt & pepper to taste.

For Your Meal:
- Arrange salmon, rice, & asparagus on a dinner plate.
- Sit down to…
- chew each bite…
- taste each bite…
- and
- Enjoy!

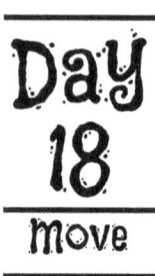

SWIM IN THE AIR...
to unfreeze and strengthen your shoulders.

Stand with feet on the floor, hip-distance apart.
Extend both arms out to each side of you,
 then alternate swinging each arm
in a half circle up, over your head ---
 straight in front of you ---
and then down across the front of you.

Do 10 strokes for each arm.
Pull in on your stomach muscles.
Dig into the floor with your toes.

Repeat for another 10 strokes for each arm.

Energizing, right?

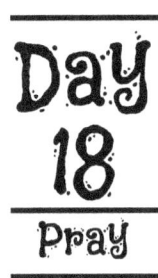

GIVE ME THE STRENGTH TO ASK FOR FORGIVENESS

Hello God,

Before I eat, remind me to sit down, and breathe.

If there is discord in my home ---- or in my life --- help me to begin the process to resolve it --- and to *wait to eat* until I am calm.

Let me recognize when I am at fault and admit it.

Let me wholly and plainly accept the blame.

Let me be willing to ask for forgiveness.

Help me to say to the one I've offended:

Yes, I_____ (gossiped about, hurt, disrespected, lied to, cheated, stole from) you. Will you forgive me?

I was selfish when I _____. Will you forgive me?

I was impatient when I _____. Will you forgive me?

I was jealous because of _____. Will you forgive me?

I was angry because I _____. Will you forgive me?

Help me not to point fingers.

Help me to admit what I did, and give the other person the freedom to not admit anything at all, even if I rationalize that he or she was primarily at fault.

Let me feel the freedom of forgiveness.

Proverbs 17:1

*Better a dry crust with peace and quiet
than a house full of feasting, with strife.*

Day 19
Think

EGGS AND DAIRY

Sometime during the last half of the 20th century, eggs became vilified. "Too much saturated fat and cholesterol in them," authorities warned. "Better to severely limit your intake of them." So you probably obediently limited your consumption of eggs, and if you craved an egg meal for breakfast, you believed the "smart" thing to do was to at least leave out the egg yolks. The word was that cholesterol lurked in the yolk, and not eating the yolk meant you were looking out for the health of your heart.

I am so, so sorry you have been led astray for so many years.

Eggs are actually very good for you --- saturated fat, cholesterol, and all.

In fact, eggs are the perfect food. (But I bet you already probably secretly believed that foods --- like eggs --- that your grandparents --- and their grandparents --- ate with no adverse health effects were probably good for you, too.)

Did you remember that your brain needs cholesterol? Your body uses cholesterol to build membranes within its cells, and eggs contain a wealth of cholesterol --- about 212 mg in each egg. Two hundred and twelve milligrams per egg is a lot compared to most other foods, but this is not a cause for worry. Just because you're eating this amount of cholesterol doesn't mean your blood level of cholesterol will increase.

What researchers learned all the way back in the 1960s is that (for most people) the amount of cholesterol you eat doesn't increase the amount of cholesterol in your blood. In 2015, the Dietary Guidelines Advisory Committee (for Americans) finally admitted that: "available evidence shows no appreciable relationship between consumption of dietary cholesterol and serum cholesterol." The committee recognized that the human livers of most people manufacture cholesterol every day --- more if a person doesn't eat enough of it and less if a person does.

The thing that researchers have come to learn and admit today is that eating eggs will actually improve your blood health. Eggs tend to pump up the presence of HDL (the good) cholesterol and will induce the transformation of LDL (the bad) cholesterol into a type that's not connected to an increased risk of heart disease.

And as for weight control, one study discovered that 3 whole eggs per day could reduce your insulin resistance, raise your HDL levels, and increased the size of LDL particles --- even if you have metabolic syndrome --- and whether or not you're a man or a woman.

Besides the fact that eggs contain healthy fats, if you want to lose weight, maintain your desired weight, and gain energy, nutritionists recommend eggs for breakfast for the following reasons:

Eggs are rich in high-quality protein.

Protein provides the building material for more than your muscles and hair. (Nevertheless, two simple ways to see if you're getting enough complete protein in your diet are to check to see if your muscles are flabby or if your hair is falling out.)

A complete protein contains twenty amino acids, some of which your body cells can manufacture. Those that your cells cannot produce are called essential, and the following nine are essential amino acids: histidine, isoleucine, leucine, lysine, methionine, phenylalanine, threonine, tryptophan and valine. All of these are necessary to include in your diet if you want your body to be able to build and rebuild the right amount of enzymes, hormones, and other body chemicals for the proper functioning of your body systems. Complete protein is also needed to build strong muscles, bones, blood, hair, and nails. Eggs provide all of these essential amino acids, so the building process is never in shut-down mode.

Eggs are filling.

Because of the high-protein content of eggs, just one or two eggs in a meal can make and keep you satisfied. In studies done comparing meals with the same calorie-content, meals containing high amounts of protein reduced appetite and increased fullness. Also, and notably, egg meals decreased the subjects' tendency to eat more during later meals.

If you're someone who obsessively daydreams about food, you'll be surprised to learn that if you consume high-protein meals your chances of daydreaming (about food!) will be reduced by 60%. Plus, high-protein meals might cause you to stay away from late-night snacking.

Eggs may boost your metabolism...

by possibly up to 80–100 calories a day!

In other words, eggs can have the same stimulating effect as the other foods (such as green tea, cinnamon, turmeric, and cayenne pepper) you read about that increase the number of calories you burn to metabolize them. *(The reason that eggs require more calories to metabolize is that all protein uses more than fat or carbohydrates.)*

Eggs are low in calories.

One egg contains about 6 grams of protein and 78 calories.

For breakfast, you might have two hard boiled eggs, a total of 156 calories.

What if you decided to scramble up two eggs (12 grams of protein) with some coconut oil? One teaspoon of coconut oil would add 39 calories, which, when added to the eggs, would total 195.

Say you add a veggie to the mix --- maybe some spinach, 1 cup chopped --- which would mean 48 more calories, plus 39 calories from another teaspoon of coconut oil if you decided to sauté the spinach.

So far this is a meal adding up to 282 calories.

Eggs:	156
Coconut Oil for the scramble:	39
Spinach:	48
Coconut Oil for the sauté:	39
Total:	282 calories

Would you like bacon with that?

Two slices:	86 calories
Total breakfast:	368 calories

And how would the calories compare if you choose to have a carbohydrate breakfast instead?

Here's a rundown for 100 grams (or one cup) of granola for different commercial brands:

Kashi Heart to Heart Honey Toasted Oat Cereal: 352 calories
Kelloggs Low Fat Granola with Raisins: 377 calories
Nature Valley Low Fat Fruit Granola: 386 calories
Quaker Simply Granola Oats, Apple, Cranberry & Almonds: 490 calories
Quaker Simply Granola Oats, Honey & Almonds: 500 calories

It's pretty obvious to see that a carbohydrate meal packs in the calories. And this same high-calorie, carbohydrate meal will not keep you feeling full and satisfied for as many hours as a protein meal will.

What about yogurt?

One of the more popular reasons people add yogurt to their diets is because of the probiotics that yogurt is supposed to contain. And an abundance of probiotics is essential for anyone who desires to lose weight and rekindle health and energy.

But with any food in today's market, it's important to check the label. Yogurt *should* contain probiotic cultures --- and the cultures are supposed to be active. But the fact is, many yogurts have had their probiotics processed right out of them. Heat-processing will kill probiotic organisms, so check to be sure. If the label states "live and active cultures," the yogurt should contain probiotics.

(It's important to always be on the lookout, though. Even if a yogurt brand claims to contain live and active cultures, it might also include thievish and unhealthy sugar or sugared fruit. One small tub --- 5.3 ounces --- of Dannon Strawberry Yogurt, for instance, might have probiotics, but it's also filled with 16 grams of sugar --- the very ingredient you're being advised to avoid. The good you're doing by eating the probiotics will be canceled out by the sugar that piggy-backs in at the same time. So please, keep your gut healthy, and you'll see that the weight you've been trying to lose for months or years will begin to melt away.)

Yogurt is high in protein, which means that it stays in your system longer. Remember that protein takes longer to digest, and is very satisfying. Being filled and satisfied is a proven way to help you stay away from bad-food snacking. Yogurt also contains a healthy portion of saturated fat. A 2012 review of clinical trials specifically showed that you can change your body composition, gain lean mass, and lose weight by eating fats in dairy products. Of course, this means dairy products without added sugar.

Butter, in moderation, is healthy, and good for your diet, too.

Who would've thought that anyone who wants to lose weight would be encouraged to eat butter?

But that's exactly what I'm encouraging you to do.

My encouragement is based on science.

Why it's good to eat butter:

In 2002, researchers at the Université Paris Sud in France tested the effect butter --- as compared to soybean oil --- would have on both lean and obese Zucker rats.

What they found was that in obese rats metabolism and fat oxidation increased when the rats were fed butter, and butter appeared to prevent fat from accumulating in adipose tissue in the long term. In the lean rats fed butter, their working muscles tended to use fats for energy.

In a famous lab experiment done by Research Diets, approximately 50,000 mice were fed a high-fat diet using lard. All of these mice gained weight, but when they were given a small amount of butyrate acid (the ester or salt of butyric acid contained in butter), the mice did not get fat and remained metabolically healthy.

Can you cook with butter?

Yes. And ghee, a more concentrated form of butter, is also a healthy option. Ghee provides slightly more butyric acid (and other short-chain saturated fats) than regular butter. And that's a good thing.

Why is butyric acid beneficial for health and weight-loss? Because test-tube and animal studies show that butyric acid, along with other short-chain fatty acids, may reduce inflammation, promote intestinal health, inhibit cancer growth, and prevent the development of insulin resistance and obesity.

Plus, butyric-acid-containing ghee is also higher in conjugated linoleic acid, that poly-unsaturated fat which may facilitate additional weight-loss. We'll talk more about conjugated linoleic acid tomorrow, and I hope you'll stay with me until then.

It's a talk that'll knock your socks off.

Today's Goal (Part A):
Consider the following protein amounts:
1 egg = 6 grams
1 container of Greek yogurt (6 ounces) = 17 grams
1 cup of Greek full-fat yogurt = 20 grams

Today's Goal (Part B):
Have an egg or two as part of a high-protein breakfast or lunch.

Day 19
Taste

FAST BRUNCH SCRAMBLE
(serves 1)

Ingredients:

2 eggs
¼ cup chopped red onions
1 cupful fresh spinach
1 tablespoon coconut oil
2 pieces paleo bacon *(nitrate- & nitrite-free; no-sugar rub)*
1 slice sprouted whole-grain bread
pink Himalayan salt & pepper to taste

Directions:

- Place the bacon into a skillet over medium-high heat & let cook.
- Plop your slice of bread into a toaster, and while toasting:

For Eggs:
- Melt 1 teaspoon of oil into a medium hot skillet.
- Chop the onions, the add to skillet and stir frequently until soft & browning at the edges.
- Break the eggs into the skillet over the onions & stir quickly, making sure the whites and yolks of the eggs are totally mixed together.
- Keep stirring until the eggs are softly scrambled, then:
- Scrape the eggs onto your breakfast plate before they dry.

For spinach:
- Melt 1 teaspoon of the coconut oil into the skillet & add the spinach.

FAST BRUNCH SCRAMBLE (serves 1)

- Stir quickly until the spinach is softened, but not overcooked.
- Transfer to the egg plate.

For toast:
- Spread the remaining coconut oil over your toast.

For your drink:
- Serve with a cup of cinnamon coffee or tea.

You can let this meal be the first meal of the day.
If you can wait until noon to eat it, all the better.

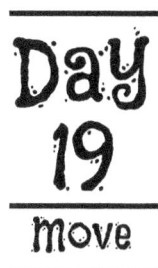

Day 19 — move

BE A "SUPERPERSON" ON A FLOOR MAT...
to strengthen your core.

Lie down on your stomach on a comfortable mat (or on a flat bed).

Reach your arms in front of you on the mat as far as you can.

Extend both legs out in back of you and point your toes.

Lift your left leg (extended with toe pointed) and hold for 5 seconds. Alternate with your right leg. Lift each leg 10 times.

Rest your legs on the mat.

Next:

With both arms extended out in front of you, elevate your left arm (palm down) and hold for 5 seconds. Alternate with your right arm. Elevate each arm 10 times --- trying to elevate it higher than your head. Do 10 lifts for each arm.

Next:

Push your stomach muscles into the floor.

Now alternate raising your right arm while you lift your left foot --- and then raise your left arm while lifting your right foot, and hold for 5 seconds.

Repeat 10 lifts for each arm-and-leg combo.

Relax and remember to breathe through your nose.

Can you "fly" 10 more strokes?

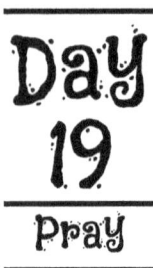

TOMORROW LEADS TO ETERNITY

Hello God,

I know that portion-size is something I ought to pay attention to when I eat.

I've been known to go overboard.

I eat too much, drink too much, sleep too much, and watch too much TV.

Moderation is a word I don't like to use. It's too old-fashioned.

Shouldn't I be taking life by the throat and squeezing out everything I can?

I mean, I only go around once, right?

But --- you say there's more enjoyment --- as well as a healthier life --- in moderation.

You say that eating too much and drinking too much will make me not only sleepier but poorer in health and in life, also.

Help me not to let my eyes be bigger than my stomach.

Help me to be moderate in the food I eat so that I may enjoy the life you've given me, and carry out with energy the work you have in mind for me to do.

Proverbs 23:20-21

*Do not join those who drink too much wine
or gorge themselves on meat,
for drunkards and gluttons become poor,
and drowsiness clothes them in rags.*

1 Corinthians 10:31

*So whether you eat or drink or whatever you do,
do it all for the glory of God.*

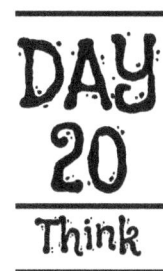

TIME FOR A TRIP TO THE RANGE
(...where the deer and the antelope play,
not where you hit golf balls...)

Surprised that we're going to talk about "meat as a choice food" in a guide which has a goal of setting you on a path to a healthy weight?

Maybe you're thinking like I did when I wandered through my sluggish and unhealthy years carrying with me the misperception that the only things meat can give you are fat and calories --- so people who want to lose weight should stay away from it.

But examining research studies and coaching others have made clear to me that meat is also an excellent source of protein, vitamins, minerals, and essential fatty acids.

The reason a section regarding meat-eating shows up here in a guide to help you lose weight, maintain your desired weight, and gain energy is because what you and I have been talking about for the last nineteen days is not a "diet," but a new way of life.

Subtle, so-called "authoritative" indoctrination over the past fifty to sixty years has left you guiltily eyeing the meat department at the grocery store, or refraining from ordering meat from any restaurant menu.

I know there are other reasons, besides "being on a diet," that people refrain from eating meat. Some believe that it is not morally right for anyone to destroy the life of an animal when other foods are available to fill up the dinner table. Around the world native cultures have a history of refusing to kill for sport, and have permitted their members to kill only if an animal was needed for sustenance. In the process of killing for sustenance, cultures sometimes observed elaborate rituals in which they thanked the animal or the source of the giver of life, and so were able to reconcile their killing with their need for food.

Others believe that animals consume or "use up" vast amounts of field grains and grasses that otherwise could be used for feeding people. (Even so, meat is a dense form of calories and eating it means that fewer alternate foods are needed to supply the right amount of calories and nutrients.)

Still others press the issue further by explaining that cows in particular produce methane, which adds to greenhouse gases.

But I am not here to discuss the ethical or environmental reasons why people refrain from eating meat.

I am here only to address those who say that eating meat will harm your health, and to address those who say that eating meat will especially hurt any attempts to lose weight.

Because the truth is just the opposite.

As you continue on your journey today, you'll find out why meat is healthy for your body, and why eating meat might be necessary for your weight-loss plan.

You read yesterday that protein provides you with a satisfying meal, better sleep, and an effective weight-loss aid.

Protein allows your body to stay alive. It gives your body structure and your hormones and enzymes tools they need to function.

You need protein to build muscles, tendons, organs, and skin.

Without proteins you wouldn't be able to digest the food you eat, your neurotransmitters wouldn't be able to communicate messages from your brain to the cells in your body, and your hormones wouldn't be able to do their jobs.

Proteins are made out of twenty smaller molecules called amino acids --- some of which your body can manufacture from other foods you eat and others of which your body cannot produce:

histidine, isoleucine, leucine, lysine, methionine, phenylalanine, threonine, tryptophan and valine. You read on Day 19 that these nine amino acids are called "essential" because it's essential to include these protein particles in your diet.

Earlier in this guide, I wrote about the importance of including enough protein in your diet --- but not too much, and it's also important to get your protein from the right sources. It's not just about quantity, it's also about quality, too.

The fact is, animal foods provide you with good-quality protein. The reason why is that animal protein contains all of the essential amino acids --- in the right proportions. After ingesting and digesting animal protein, your body can go right to work satisfying your hunger, then constructing, communicating, transporting... and otherwise keeping you alive.

Four excellent animal sources of protein include fish, eggs, dairy products, and meat.

Meats have been demonized over the last fifty to sixty years because of their content of saturated fat. But what medical professionals didn't understand, failed to recognize, or were prevented from publicly acknowledging, is that meat contains all three types of fatty acids --- saturated, mono-unsaturated, and poly-unsaturated --- that are extremely important for health.

For instance, red meat, pork, and poultry contain stearic acid (a saturated fat), oleic acid (a mono-unsaturated fat), linoleic acid (a poly-unsaturated fat), and conjugated linoleic acid (*a natural and healthy* trans-fat). All four are beneficial to specific areas of your body and brain.

Stearic acid is a long-chain fatty acid made up of 18 carbon atoms with no double bonds. Although it is classified as a saturated fatty acid (SFA), data accumulated during the past fifty years indicate that stearic acid is quite unique. Unlike other long-chain SFAs --- such as palmitic acid (containing 16 carbons) and myristic acid (containing 14 carbons) which increase blood cholesterol levels --- stearic acid has been shown to have a neutral effect on total blood cholesterol levels, as well as a neutral effect on low density lipoproteins (the bad cholesterol). Because of these two factors, stearic acid will not increase your chances of cardiovascular disease (CVD). What will increase your chances of CVD is inflammation caused by stress, added sugars, or refined carbohydrates in your diet.

Fats that are rich in stearic acid include mutton tallow (made by cutting up the hard, white, fatty layer surrounding a sheep's organs, heating these fatty pieces until they melt, filtering the resulting liquid, and then allowing the liquid to cool so that it resolidifies back into a solid), beef tallow, pig lard, and butter. Only 8% of the fat in a skinless, roasted chicken would be stearic acid --- whereas the stearic acid in beef would be twice as much --- about 16% of its total fat.

The first point to realize is that a piece of meat is not 100% fat. A lean cut of grass-fed beef, for instance, might contain only 15% fat. (On the other hand, some say that to make the juiciest, most flavorful burgers, you need to use ground beef that is 30% fat.) And while many people believe that 100% of the fat in beef is saturated, the truth is that even in the tallow, only 50% is saturated, while 42% is mono-unsaturated, and 4% is poly-unsaturated. (The remaining 4% is made up of other lipids and healthy conjugated linoleic acid.)

Within the 42% of mono-unsaturated fat, you can find the omega-9 fatty acid which you were introduced to as oleic acid. This is the same omega-9 fatty acid you (hopefully by now!) are consuming in olive oil, avocados, macadamia nuts, and pecans. Oleic acid is known for not only lowering your blood pressure to within a healthy range, but it's also known to increase fat-burning. And one of the reasons you're reading this guide is to find out ways you can increase fat-burning, right? So why not include foods in your diet that can help you do that?

Oleic acid does more than increase the fat-burning potential of your cells, by the way. It works to keep you healthy by preventing free-radical damage in your cells, by preventing Type-2 Diabetes, and by protecting your digestive tract from developing sores or ulcers. Oleic acid --- or omega-9 --- also generates the protective sheath called myelin around the nerves of your brain. When your brain is healthy, you feel better and have a better mindset to continue working on your weight-loss goals.

The truth is, your body can make omega-9 fats. They are not essential like the omega-6 (linoleic acid) and omega-3 (alpha-linolenic) fats are. But you can reduce the stress on your body and mind by ingesting portions of oleic acid in your diet.

Remember that foods high in oleic acid (which is present in mono-unsaturated fat) include olive oil, avocados, macadamia nuts, pecans, almonds, cashews, hazelnuts, and pistachios. Fish, eggs, and dairy also contain mono-unsaturated fat (almost 50% of the fat in an egg is oleic acid; milk fat is 25% oleic acid). And now you know that the fat in meat contains portions of oleic acid, too.

It's within the 4% poly-unsaturated fat in beef and other meats that you find something unique --- a type of fatty acid called conjugated linoleic acid (CLA). This is a poly-unsaturated fat that contains both *cis* and *trans* double bonds --- meaning that CLA is technically a trans-fat. But this is the type of trans-fat we spoke of earlier --- the type that occurs naturally in many healthy foods such as grass-fed sheep, beef, and raw dairy products that come from grass-fed cattle --- and the type that is good for you.

Did you know that as little as 0.5% of CLA in your diet could reduce cancerous tumors by up to 50% in certain places in your body?

CLA can also minimize asthma, insulin resistance, and food-induced allergic reactions.

CLA can affect the composition of your body!

CLA changes the composition of your body by lowering your body fat, increasing your metabolic rate, and has an even more significant effect if you eat it regularly and exercise, too. (Day 20 references at the end of the book will verify these statements.) The added benefit is that while your body fat is being lowered, CLA prevents muscle-loss.

Since CLA cannot be manufactured in the human body, you must get it from your diet, and high-quality sources like grass-fed sheep or beef and raw milk from grass-fed cattle are the sources to choose.

Grass-fed beef also tends to contain a higher proportion of cholesterol-neutral stearic acid, rather than the type of fatty acids that raise LDL cholesterol. Several studies suggest that if you eat meat from animals fed a grass-based diet (rather than a grain-fed diet) you would be able to absorb more Vitamins A and E from the other foods you eat, and also increase the activity of cancer-fighting antioxidants (like glutathione and superoxide dismutase) in your system.

Meat (included with poultry and fish in the USDA MyPlate's protein group) is healthy because it's made up of not only protein but also of some other unique ingredients that plants don't contain:

- *Meat contains Vitamin-B12*
  Vitamin-B12 is an essential nutrient needed for many functions throughout your body, including the production of red blood cells, DNA, and RNA. It helps your nerves to function smoothly and your body to metabolize nutrients so you can produce energy.
  Because of its role in red blood cell production, Vitamin-B12 deficiency can lead to a number of problems, including anemia.
  Specific symptoms of Multiple Sclerosis and Alzheimer's Disease (like fatigue, mental confusion, numbness, tingling of the hands and feet) might also show up if you are deficient in Vitamin-B12, since B12 assists in the metabolism of the fatty acids that protect the myelin sheath around your nerves.
  If you have weakened muscles, are feeling run-down, nervous, cranky, or depressed, you may be lacking Vitamin-B12, and eating meat may help.
  According to MayoClinic.com, the recommended daily amount of Vitamin-B12 is 2.4 micrograms for adults, 2.6 micrograms for pregnant women and 2.8 micrograms for lactating women. In general, consuming Vitamin-B12 in foods such as meat, dairy products, and eggs will enable you to meet your Vitamin-B12 requirements. The National Institutes of Health Office of Dietary Supplements

recommends to people who are at risk for developing a deficiency --- such as older adults (Vitamin-B12 absorption decreases as you age) and vegetarians --- take Vitamin-B12 supplements.

- *Meat contains creatine*
  Creatine builds an energy reserve in the brain and muscles.

- *Meat contains carnosine*
  Carnosine prevents numerous degenerative processes and serves as a significant antioxidant.

- *Meat contains Heme iron*
  Heme iron is the only type of iron your body can use, and it only comes from animal creatures which have protein hemoglobins built into their structures. Plants are not comprised of hemoglobins. Hemoglobins are only contained in meat, poultry, and fish.
  Iron is necessary for building oxygen-carrying red blood cells. Without enough red blood cells, you become fatigued and can develop anemia. A woman, especially, requires more iron in her diet due to the loss of blood during menstruation. If a woman is a meat-eater, she usually doesn't need to worry about insufficient iron.
  Iron also strengthens skin, hair, and nails.

- *Meat contains zinc*
  Zinc is a mineral important for hair, skin, and nails, as well as wound-healing, healthy eyesight, and hormones. (Are you losing your hair or really susceptible to colds? A zinc deficiency may be your problem.)

- *Meat contains L-arginine*
  L-arginine is an amino acid that can reduce body fat and works to keep your appetite in check.

- *Meat contains leucine*
  Leucine helps produce human growth hormone and can help regulate your blood sugar. If you're wanting to lose weight or prevent growing a "spare tire," eat some leucine! Regulating your blood sugar helps control the fat around your middle.

- *Meat affects testosterone levels*
  Research shows that eating meat can increase testosterone levels which, even for women, is a good thing. A decrease in testosterone levels often leads to depression, muscle weakness, lower self-esteem, and increased weight.

Meat that's best is the kind that's cut from grass-fed animals. Don't be shy about asking your butcher where your beef comes from. The best option for your health (and for losing weight) would be to eat the meat from animals organically-fed and pasture-raised, not from animals raised in confined-animal-feeding operations (CAFOs). Pasture-raised animals are usually least-exposed to antibiotics and have been found to have higher nutritional value.

Organ meats, like the liver and heart, for instance, are packed with healthy fats (including omega-3s), proteins, vitamins (including B12 that's so important for blood health and energy), and minerals.

Some people think that because the liver works as a digestive filtering system for animals as well as humans, toxins end up being stored within it. But even though the liver is a complex machine that metabolizes food, chemically alters it, and then directs it to needy places throughout the body, it is a nutrient-packed food to eat.

So, why was it that you wanted to stay away from eating meat?

While you're thinking, I just want to remind you: You must have enough protein in your diet, but not too much (like Goldilocks), because too much protein...can cause kidney damage...leach minerals from bones...cause dehydration...and has even been shown to be a contributing factor in the growth of cancer cells.

- The DRI (Dietary Reference Intake) says you should consume 0.36 grams of protein per pound of body weight, or 0.8 grams per kilogram. This amounts to 56 grams per day for the average sedentary man and 46 grams per day for the average sedentary woman. If you have a regular exercise regimen (lap swimming, running, or gym workouts at least 3x week), or are pregnant, then you need 25 to 50 percent more than this.

So picture this as you plan your daily intake:

- The amount of protein in 3 ounces of chicken breast: 26 grams
- The amount of protein in 3 ounces of beef steak: 22 grams
- The amount of protein in 3 ounces of wild-caught salmon: 17 grams
- The amount of protein in 3 ounces of bacon (about 1 ½ slice): 9.9 grams
- The amount of protein in 1 boiled egg: 6 grams
- The amount of protein in 1 cup of Greek full-fat yogurt: 20 grams

Would you like a quick way to visualize how much protein might be the right amount your body needs at each meal?

If you are a woman: the *size of your palm* can indicate the size (or amount) of protein that might be right for you. *One palm-sized portion* of eggs, fish, seafood, poultry, or red meat should satisfy and fortify you.

(Please test yourself in this. There are times your body may require more protein --- after strenuous exercise, for example --- and there are other times you may need less.)

If you are a man, the *size of two of your palms* can indicate the size (or amount) of protein that might be right for you. *Two palm-sized portions* of eggs, fish, seafood, poultry, or red meat should satisfy and fortify you.

(Please test yourself in this. There are times your body may require more protein --- after strenuous exercise, for example --- and there are other times you may need less.)

If you are a vegetarian, you should know that:

It's more challenging to get all twenty amino acids in the right proportions from vegetarian sources because there are only two vegetarian foods that provide all of the essentials: hemp seed and quinoa. One ounce of hemp seeds (about 3 tablespoons) will give you 11 grams of protein, or approximately 20% of your daily complete protein requirement if you are an average sedentary man. One cup of quinoa, on the other hand, contains only 8 grams of protein.

Some nutritionists suggest combining one incomplete protein food with another that contains the missing amino acid(s). For instance, rice protein is high in the sulfur-containing amino acids cysteine and methionine, but low in lysine (often the amino acid that many vegan eaters fail to consume). Plant foods high in lysine include legumes (peas, beans, lentils, peanuts), pistachios, and pumpkin seeds. So you'd consume a complete protein by combining rice with one of the above ingredients. But these come with a few of their own problems.

The skins of beans and other legumes (as well as portions of nuts and seeds) contain two types of toxic compounds known as phytates and lectins. These anti-nutrients are meant to protect beans/legumes, nuts, and seeds from invading microorganisms, pests, and insects as they grow. But these compounds can be very harmful to humans.

When a human consumes foods high in phytates (or phytic acid), that person will absorb less of the life-affirming minerals that he or she needs, like iron, zinc, manganese, and calcium. (Phytates occur in high percentages in grains, too, by the way.)

As for the lectins in beans, legumes, grains, nuts, and seeds, not all of them are bad. But some are related directly to inflammation. They will attach themselves to your cell membranes and cause great harm to your health. (Dr. Mercola advises that if you are struggling with an autoimmune disease, you may benefit from a lectin-restricted diet.)

Plus, lectins are a hidden (but measurable) reason for weight gain. Even though your body will resist digesting them, they are able to change the environment of your gut biome by allowing more "bad" (rather than "good") bacteria to grow or flourish. And maintaining a balanced gut biome is essential if you want to have any hope for healthy weight-loss and maintaining a healthy weight.

Dr. Steven Gundry, author of the book *The Plant Paradox: The Hidden Dangers in 'Healthy' Foods That Cause Disease and Weight Gain* (2017), says that lectins can lead to leaky gut syndrome because they interfere with the absorption of nutrients across your intestinal wall.

One of the ways to mitigate the dangerous effects of phytates and lectins is to soak your beans and legumes before cooking them, or buy brands that are sold pre-soaked. Then cook them thoroughly, until they are very soft. Soaking and cooking in this way will also make beans and legumes (as well as nuts and seeds) more digestible.

Research has found that eating a strictly plant-based diet can put you at risk of subclinical protein malnutrition, which means you're also likely not getting enough dietary sulfur. And you may become deficient in omega-3s, which are best obtained from fish, meats, and other animal protein sources.

A quick review for vegetarians:

The 4 essential amino acids missing from many plant foods are lysine, tryptophan, methionine, and phenylalanine.

- *Plant foods high in lysine include*:
  legumes, peas, beans, lentils, peanuts, pistachios, and pumpkin seeds.
- *Plant foods high in tryptophan include*:
  Butternut squash seeds, sea vegetables (kelp, seaweed, and spirulina), cucumber, whole wheat, walnuts, potatoes, cauliflower, and leafy greens.
- *Plant foods high in methionine include*:
  Nuts (almonds, walnuts, hazelnuts, pine nuts), seeds (sunflower, pumpkin, pistachio, sesame), grains (brown rice, barley, oats, whole wheat), spinach, buckwheat, watercress, and purslane.
- *Plant foods high in phenylalanine*:
  Almonds, pecans, pumpkin seeds, sesame seeds, peanuts, bananas, avocadoes, brewer's yeast, corn, lima beans, whole grains, chickpeas, and lentils.

If you want to choose vegetarian protein sources for your diet, mix and match those foods listed above.

One common approach is to combine grains (brown rice, oats, whole wheat, or rye) with beans or lentils. Grains contain the cysteine and methionine that beans and lentils lack, and beans and lentils contain the lysine that grains lack.

Here are nutritionally recommended combos for vegetarian-sourced protein:

- Brown rice with lentils
- Brown rice with black beans
- Brown rice with split pea soup
- Black bean soup with whole wheat bread
- Peanut butter on whole wheat bread

Today's Goal:

Feel free to include a serving of lamb, beef, or chicken at lunch or dinner. *Avoid processed meats like bologna, sausage, or bacon that contain artificial preservatives, chemical fillers, and added sugars.*

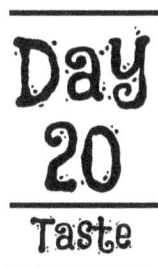

CHOICE CHICKEN DINNER
(serves 2)

Ingredients:

1 chicken breast, bone-in
2 small sweet potatoes
2 stalks broccoli (about 2 cups, chopped)
coconut oil
pink Himalayan salt
pepper
garlic powder
paprika
1-2 tablespoons butter

Directions:

For Sweet Potatoes:
- Clean each potato with a vegetable brush.
- Use your hands to massage coconut oil around each potato & wrap into aluminum foil.
  (Now rub the coconut oil all over your hands…& face, if you're daring! Coconut oil is an effective skin cleanser & conditioner.)
- Bake at 350 degrees for 1 hour.
- When done, remove potatoes from foil, cut each in half and serve with butter.

For Chicken:
- Pre-heat oven to 350 degrees.
- Spread a teaspoon or so of coconut oil on the bottom of a Pyrex dish big enough for your piece of chicken.

- Remove the skin from the chicken breast, then slice into the thick portion of the breast so that the meat can be splayed with a piece of the meat on either side of the bone.
- Rub coconut oil all over the chicken breast, then sprinkle with salt, pepper, garlic powder, & paprika to taste.
- Place chicken bone-side up in baking dish.
- Bake for 30-35 minutes, or until chicken is nicely browned.
- Cut into the meat to make sure the interior of the chicken is cooked thoroughly *(the meat should be white, not pink)*.

For Broccoli:
- Clean and remove any hard exterior covering from the stalks.
- Chop the stems and heads into smaller pieces.
- Add broccoli to a cooking pot. Cover the bottom of the pot with purified water and cook on medium heat for about 10 minutes.

    (Don't put too much water into the pot that you'll have to throw away, but

    don't put too little water either because the pot will burn. Experiment with

    ½ cup water first, and see if you're able to cook with this amount until the broccoli's soft but still crunchy. Of course, you can also steam the broccoli for

    10 minutes instead.)
- When done, dress with 1 pat of butter, pink Himalayan sea salt and black pepper to taste.

When Ready:
- Arrange chicken, sweet potatoes, and broccoli on plates, and place on your table.
- Before sitting down, breathe in and out deeply.
- Sit down, chew, and…
  -Enjoy!

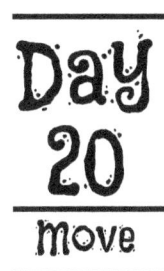

SQUAT...
to strengthen your legs and your core.

Stand with feet on the floor, hip-distance apart.

Now bend at the knees with your buttocks extended back.

Try to squat down so that your upper legs are parallel to the floor.

It's okay to push out your arms for balance as you squat down.

Your arms will naturally come up into a bend.

At each squat, dig into the floor with your toes for balance.

Do 10 squats.

Rest.

Then repeat 2 more times.

Next week up the number to 15, and repeat 3 times.

When you finish, feel the rush.

Enjoy!

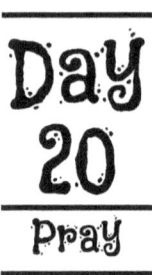

Day 20 — Pray

EXPLAIN IT TO ME, PLEASE.

Hello God,

You're the creator and engineer of my body's machinery.

You know what kind of fuel --- and how much --- my body "machine" --- requires to operate well.

Impress upon me that too much protein can clog up the engine.

Continue to give me the power to say "yes" to the foods and drinks that bring life, and the power to say "no" to the foods and drinks which can destroy life.

Please give me the desire, strength, and knowledge to protect and maintain my body-engine.

Romans 14:2-4

*One person's faith allows them to eat anything,
but another, whose faith is weak, eats only vegetables.
The one who eats everything
must not treat with contempt the one who does not,
and the one who does not eat everything
must not judge the one who does,
for God has accepted them.
Who are you to judge someone else's servant?
To their own master, servants stand or fall.
And they will stand,
for the Lord is able to make them stand.*

1 Corinthians 6:19-20

*Do you not know
that your bodies are temples of the Holy Spirit,
who is in you,
whom you have received from God?
You are not your own;
you were bought at a price.
Therefore, honor God with your bodies.*

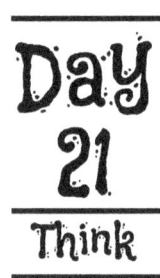

GRAINS, GLUTEN, & CARBS THAT COUNT

If you did what I did for years --- if you cut out as many fats as you could and filled up on carbohydrates instead --- if you ate muffins or cereal for breakfast instead of bacon and eggs (because you believed you were protecting your heart) --- scientists owe you and me an apology. They are finally admitting what most current epidemiological and clinical trial data show: That cardiovascular disease actually worsens with increased carbohydrates (especially sugar), or shows no improvement at all!

The second consequence of eating more carbohydrates in place of fats was more fat around my belly! Did you experience the same phenomenon?

You already know that if you want to lose weight, maintain a healthy weight, and gain energy, you need to eliminate refined carbohydrates --- and all sugars are refined carbohydrates. They'll deny you your goals every step of the way.

Refined carbohydrates include and are found in table sugar, syrups, sweeteners, soft drinks, jellies, jams, candies, sugared cereals, cookies, and cakes.

But did you know that limiting other refined carbohydrates would be great for your health and your waistline, too?

Other refined carbohydrates include:
- White flour (used to coat and season foods like chicken and fish)
- White bread and toast

- Bagels
- Fat-free snacks (like chips and crackers)
- White bread pizza
- White pasta
- White rice
- Muffins

On the other hand, whole, fiber-rich carbohydrates are needed in a healthy diet, and below you're going to see why.

But first, are you wondering exactly which carbohydrates are whole, fiber-rich, and healthy for you?

And maybe you're also wondering exactly which ones help you lose weight (I know that's why you've stayed with me until this 21st day). So I'm going to tell you.

Grains are the edible, dry seeds from plants like corn (maize), rice and wheat. Grain-products filled the base of the United States Department of Agriculture "Food Guide Pyramid" for more than two decades. Beginning in 1992, the US government was recommending that the majority of your diet should consist of grains. Currently throughout the world, corn, rice, and wheat now provide more food energy than any other food group --- but mostly in their unnatural, refined state.

The world seems to not be aware, however, that the USDA 1992 Food Guide Pyramid was replaced by a new 2005 MyPyramid, which was then replaced by the 2011 ChooseMyPlate food guide. The USDA now recommends fewer grains and more vegetables. (Sadly, the USDA still recommends low levels of saturated fats while at the same time recommending dangerously high levels of poly-unsaturated fats. Hopefully, the USDA will change its mind once more to reflect current science, and recommend that healthy saturated fats be reinserted back into your diet.)

How about you? Should you get your energy from corn, wheat, and rice? Are these safe to consume from any source, and in any form? Is it really so important to stay away from refined grains --- or grains with their germ and fiber removed --- such as refined corn, white bread or white rice? White bread is everywhere, after all. If restaurants and shops continually offer it, can it really be so bad? And how about white rice? Consuming white rice has become even more popular now that sushi is a favorite exotic food. Surely the Japanese know what they're doing and wouldn't lead us down an unhealthy path. White bread and white rice have to be good for us, right?

No!

Because white bread, white rice, and refined corn are milled to remove the valuable germ (containing healthy fat and protein) and friendly fiber. What's left is mostly starch --- a refined carbohydrate that causes sticky build-up in your blood vessels and promotes inflammation throughout your body.

Further problems come with genetically modified grains.

Since 1996 the US has allowed the use of genetically-modified (GMO) corn, and in 2014, according to the USDA, 93% of (field) corn crops planted in the United States contained GMOs. (GMO seeds now produce more than 90 percent of soy and canola crops, as well.) So if you're eating foods like commercial cornbread, corn flake cereal, or corn pasta with the bran and germ removed, you're probably eating GMO refined corn.

Can you avoid refined GMO corn?

You can if you consume organically-grown corn products instead of conventionally grown ones --- and if you make sure their labels say: whole grain (meaning that no processing has removed the bran or the germ). Buying products labeled 100% Organic, Certified Organic, and USDA Organic is usually the easiest way to identify and avoid genetically modified ingredients.

The United States and Canadian governments do NOT allow companies to label products "100% Organic" or "Certified Organic" if they contain genetically modified foods.

What about wheat? Are the following two doctors and one popular diet mentioned below wrong when they say you should avoid it entirely if you want to lose weight?

Dr. Mark Hyman, author of the New York Times best-selling book *The Blood Sugar Solution (2014)*, explains that decades of cross-breeding and hybridization have produced a shorter, stockier "dwarf wheat" (which some have been known to call *frankenwheat*), and this dwarf wheat makes up almost all of the wheat consumed in the United States today. The problem with it, Dr. Hyman explains, is that "it also contains high levels of a 'super starch' called amylopectin A, which excels at making both Cinnabons and bellies swell."

Dr. William Davis agrees that if you want to get rid of your belly fat, you should forgo wheat altogether. In his book *Wheat Belly: Lose the Wheat, Lose the Weight and Find Your Path Back to Health (2011)*, Dr. Davis describes how our current shorter, fatter wheat contains different glutens that many humans are intolerant to. Plus, Dr. Davis warns, wheat is addictive.

The popular Paleo Diet recommends eliminating almost all grains completely from your diet in order to lose weight --- and to stay healthy --- because of the dangers of the lectins, phytates, and gluten they contain. As a result, many people all over the world are now avoiding grains because they believe all grains are unhealthy.

> **The truth is, if you eliminate grains from your diet, you *will* lose weight.**

BUT, whole grains are vital components of a healthy diet. Grains provide a feeling of satisfaction when you eat them. Many people find that they continue to feel hungry --- no matter how much food from other food groups is eaten --- if they don't eat a certain amount of grain products. If you are not allergic or sensitive to gluten, even wholegrain wheat (organic) is good for you because it contains numerous proteins, fiber, vitamins, and minerals. The reason why whole grains are better than refined is that they are resistant to "quick digestion," which means that your body doesn't have to produce extra amounts of insulin and your blood sugar levels remain balanced.

> **A way to stay on the healthy side of the grain argument:**

Choose whole grains. This means cooking or baking with corn, rice, and wheat that contain the germ plus the bran. It involves selecting brown, black, or wild rice instead of white, brown breads instead of white, refined ones, and choosing organically-grown grains rather than conventionally grown grains, especially for wheat and corn.

Many people do find that when they eliminate gluten from their diet, they lose weight without even having to think about it. So I would recommend that while you are trying to lose weight, you eliminate as much gluten as possible.

My suggestion is to listen to your body. If a particular food or drink gives you a headache or a runny nose or leaves you feeling bloated or extra-tired, don't consume it. Whether it's organic wheat or not, listen to your body.

Below are grains that are good for your diet & good for you.

Also listed are the reasons why.

The first 5 are gluten-free, and the last 2 contain gluten. (And you should know that while many people have personally testified that going gluten-free has helped to streamline their waistlines, there are no current studies to back up their claim.)

What often happens for most dieters (and I'm not saying this is you...) is that they'll swap a wheat product for a non-gluten millet or rice product, and the non-gluten swap contains more sugar and more of the wrong kind of fat (to make up for the lost taste of wheat) than the gluten product they're swapping. They consume more bad calories, and they could end up gaining weight!

Reading ingredient labels is important. As you do so, keep in mind what you're learning in this guide. Try to include all whole grains in your diet (from the list below) and eliminate processed sugars and processed fats.

1. *Brown Rice (Gluten-Free)*: Can help stabilize your blood sugar because it's high in fiber. It has a wealth of antioxidants and is an excellent source of manganese as well as a good source of magnesium and selenium. Because of the B-Vitamins contained in brown rice, you can eat it as a stress-reducing food.

2. *Millet (Gluten-Free):* This grain is a good source of manganese, phosphorous, and magnesium. It can help with the development and repair of your cells, it can protect against breast cancer, and it can also help keep away gallstones.

3. *Oats (Gluten-Free):* Help to fight infection and stabilize your blood sugar.

4. *Quinoa (Gluten-Free):* Though quinoa is actually a seed, it's generally considered to be a grain. The great benefit of quinoa is that it is a complete protein. (However, while quinoa does have all the essential amino acids, it contains minimal amounts in each portion, and would require buckets of consumption to equal the amount of protein in a serving of eggs, meat or even legumes.) Quinoa is also high in Vitamin-E and calcium.

5. *Buckwheat (Gluten-Free):* Buckwheat, in fact, is not a type of wheat at all, but a relative of rhubarb. The Japanese use buckwheat to make soba noodles, but you can also eat the seeds by either grinding them into flour (for gluten-free pancakes!) or cooking the hulled kernels (called "groats") into a breakfast porridge. Buckwheat is also good for blood-sugar control and is known to prevent gallstones.

6. *Whole Wheat (Not Gluten-Free):* Rich in proteins and B-Vitamins. It is also a good source of Vitamin-E.

7. *Barley (Not Gluten-Free):* A terrific source of fiber and selenium (necessary for proper function of your thyroid). Barley contains usable amounts of phosphorous, copper, manganese, and barley in your diet can prevent gallstones.

How many grams of carbohydrates should you have a day?

100 to 150 grams a day will provide you with the fiber and nutrients you need to stay healthy while you are losing weight.

By contrast, the *Dietary Guidelines for Americans* recommends that if you're consuming a standard 2,000-calorie daily diet, you should eat 225 to 325 grams of total carbohydrates per day, adding up to roughly half of your daily calories. (Total carbohydrates wouldn't just include the carbs in grains, but also the carbs in fruits and vegetables, and whatever sweeteners you're using.)

You've probably guessed that eliminating all refined grains from your diet --- saying "no" to cakes, donuts, cookies, white bread, refined-grain crackers, muffins, rolls, white rice, most snack chips, and most packaged cereals --- would be a healthy action to take --- and would add power to your ability to lose weight. Can you do it? Can you choose whole-wheat bread, whole grain oats, millet, quinoa, brown rice and homemade popcorn instead of other versions that contain half the nutrients and cause twice the havoc in your system?

If you're not ready to take this drastic (but very freeing step!) can you at least make a pact with yourself to decrease the amount of refined grains you eat each day?

And while you're decreasing the amount of refined grains, will you at the same time make a pact to increase the amount of *good* fats in your diet? If so, you will find yourself very satisfied.

Counting grams of proteins, carbohydrates, and fiber is a healthier way to consider your daily consumption of food rather than counting calories.

For instance:
- One slice of Ezekiel sprouted grain bread (grains include: wheat, barley, beans, lentils, millet, and spelt):
    protein = 4 grams; carbs = 15 grams; fiber = 3 grams
- One packet of plain instant oats:
    proteins = 5.4 grams; carbs = 19 grams; fiber = 3.7 grams
- One cup of cooked oatmeal:
    protein = 6 grams; carbs = 32 grams; fiber = 8.2 grams
- One cup of cooked bulgur:
    protein = 5.6 grams; carbs = 34 grams; fiber = 8 grams
- One cup of cooked millet:
    protein = 6 grams; carbs = 41 grams; fiber = 2 grams
- One cup of cooked quinoa:

protein = 8 grams; carbs = 39 grams; fiber = 5 grams
- One cup of buckwheat flour:
  protein = 15 grams; carbs = 85 grams; fiber = 12 grams
- One cup of cooked whole-wheat pasta:
  protein = 7.5 grams; carbs = 37 grams; fiber = 6 grams
- One cup of whole-grain brown rice:
  protein = 5 grams; carbs = 51 grams; fiber = 3.5 grams
- One 7-inch organic, whole grain corn tortilla:
  protein = 1 gram; carbs = 8 grams; fiber = 1.5 grams

The other type of carbohydrate that you should be aware of is that found in starchy vegetables, beans and legumes. For instance:

- One cup of green peas:
  protein = 8.5 grams; carbs = 25 grams; fiber = 8.5 grams
- One cup of sweet potato, baked in skin:
  protein = 11 grams; carbs = 34 grams; fiber = 6.5 grams
- One cup of cooked chickpeas:
  protein = 14.5 grams; carbs = 45 grams; fiber = 12.5 grams
- One cup of black beans:
  protein = 15 grams; carbs = 40 grams; fiber = 15 grams

And who would've thought that being healthy might involve a little math…?

Today's Goal (a boosted effort on Day 21!):

Will you decide today to limit your total intake of *total carbohydrates from grains, starchy vegetables, beans and legumes* to 100 grams a day (if you're a female) and 150 grams a day (if you're a male)? Test to see what 100 or 150 grams look like.

This means that --- if you're eating packaged foods and cereals --- you've got to read the packaging labels and take note of what one serving is.

Does this sound like too much work? Acquiring a new skill is always more challenging in the beginning. But with repetition, the doing becomes easier. And pretty soon, you'll guess pretty accurately how many grams of carbohydrates are contained in the amounts of food set before you.

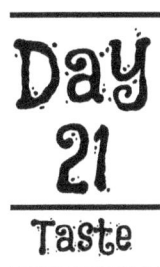

GLUTEN-FREE PANCAKES
(makes about 9-10 pancakes, or about 3 servings)

Ingredients:

1 egg
1/2 cup cassava flour
1/2 cup buckwheat flour
1/4 cup coconut flour
1/4 cup almond flour
1 teaspoon baking powder
1 teaspoon baking soda
1 1/2 cups buttermilk
OR: *To make dairy-free "buttermilk": add 1 tablespoon of lemon juice to 1 1/2 cups of coconut milk (unsweetened) & let sit for 5 minutes before using.*
1 cup blueberries
4 tablespoons coconut oil
maple syrup
1/4 cup freshly ground flaxseed

Directions:

- Scramble the *egg* in a large bowl.
- Add 3 tablespoons of *coconut oil*.
- Mix in the *buttermilk* or soured *coconut milk*.
- Drop in the *berries*.
- In a separate bowl, combine *cassava flour, buckwheat flour, coconut flour, almond flour, baking powder & baking soda*.

- Add the dry mix to the *milk/egg/berry* bowl.
- Stir evenly just until you make sure the wet and dry ingredients are combined; don't over-stir.

- Melt enough coconut oil into a medium-hot pan or griddle so that pancakes will not stick.
- Use a soup ladle to drop portions of pancake mixture onto the pan.
- Cook until bubbles form on the top side of the cakes.
- Turn over with a spatula.
- Cook the remaining side until brown.

This recipe makes about 3 servings. The size of your pancakes will depend on how much pancake mixture you put in your ladle. I usually form them to be about 4 inches wide.
Pancakes cook better if all ingredients are room temperature.

- When done, sprinkle the ground flaxseed and drizzle 1 or 2 tablespoons of hot natural maple syrup over the cakes. Serve with sauteed spinach or green beans.
- Enjoy!

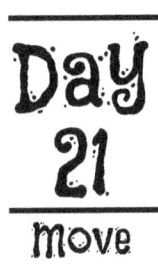

Day 21
move

OVERALL EXERCISE...
to strengthen and energize your shoulders, legs, and core.
(*Originated by Dr. Zach Bush*)

1. Complete 10 squats as you did yesterday.
2. After your first set of squats, stand up straight and extend your arms straight out in front of you until they're parallel with the floor.
   Lift and lower each straight arm from waist to shoulder height, 10 times, alternating arms.
   After your set of arm raises, lower your arms and hands and let them rest in front of you.
3. Now form a fist with each hand.
   Swing your left arm in a wide half-circle out to the left side and over your head --- as you swing your right arm in a wide half-circle out to the right side and over your head.
   Make sure both arms meet fist-to-fist at the end of your straightened arms above your head.
   Swing your straightened arms back down in front of you and touch fist-to-fist in front of your groin.
   Do 10 full circles.
4. Next, bend your arms and raise them to shoulder height.
   Then from shoulder height, reach both of your arms to the ceiling.
   Dig into the floor with your toes for balance and tighten your stomach muscles.
   Reach up 10 times.

When you finish these four sets, feel the rush.

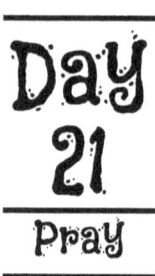

LET ME BEGIN AGAIN...?

I've only just begun, God.

Health surely is a journey. And now I see that for some people like me the progress isn't straightforward.

Learning a new skill takes time because to really learn it you've got to practice it, too.

And teaching myself to crave things that are good for me may demand lots of patience and perseverance. Please give me the patience to try (at least 12 times!) the foods or movements that are good for me.

Let me continue to begin each day, God, in conversation with you.

Remind me always that you are a God of new beginnings.

Lamentations 3:22-23
Because of the Lord's great love we are not consumed,
for his compassions never fail.
They are new every morning;
great is your faithfulness.

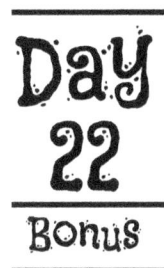

ONE MIGHTY TOOL TO RESET MIND AND BODY

This last tool has been kept a secret for far too long, and I've been yearning to reveal it to you. I was keen to disclose it at the beginning of your journey with me but wasn't sure you were ready. How do I know that you're ready now? Because I believe that your time with me has prepared you to answer the following question correctly:

Why do you choose the foods you eat, the thoughts you think, and the ways you move your body?

If you were fully engaged with me during the last twenty-one days, you have come to understand that part of the answer involves habits and hormones.

Habits and hormones are two of the most dominant influencers in your life. Many people think that once set, they can't be changed.

But on this Bonus Day, I'm here to emphasize again that they can be changed --- and to give you one more potent tool to use.

Intermittent Fasting is such a tool.

With it, you can break away from unhealthy eating habits and reset the influence of powerful hormones --- once and for all.

Intermittent means doing something on and off, or in intervals.

Fasting means to go without food for a period of time.

Intermittent Fasting, then, is to go without food for periods of time, on and off, or in intervals. It means to refrain from eating for certain days of the week, or for certain extended hours of each day.

Why is Intermittent Fasting helpful for losing weight, maintaining a desired weight, and gaining energy?

When you consume regular meals throughout a 24-hour day, you're most likely consuming food in the form of carbohydrates or sugars --- because carbohydrates and sugars make up the major portion of the diet for most Americans. Your body will naturally use energy gained from these readily-available carbohydrate/sugar calories because your body prefers to burn sugar as energy before any other source. But when you refrain from eating for increased amounts of time, your body doesn't have a freshly ingested meal to access for energy. The longer you deprive your body of carbohydrates, the more it will search for fat stored in your body's cells to use for the energy it needs.

And, of course, that's one of the reasons why you're here. To burn fat.

Intermittent fasting will help you do just that.

Intermittent fasting works because it limits calories naturally. Whether you choose to refrain from eating for 24 hours every few days or to fast for 16 hours every day, you will eventually be lowering the number of calories you eat during the week. Normally, by incorporating the kinds of foods into your diet that we've talked about during our past twenty-one days together, fewer calories in should mean fewer pounds on your body.

You can practice Intermittent Fasting a few different ways:

Refrain from eating for 24 hours 2-3 times a week.

I personally don't find this option practical. Fasting for a full 24 hours for two or three times a week can be confining when social events are on my calendar and those events center around meals. I'll either have to skip my plan to fast or skip the event.

On the other hand, the second type of Intermittent Fasting is:

Refrain from eating for 12 to 16 hours every day.

This style I find I can incorporate into my daily schedule because it's easy to just skip breakfast.

For instance: if I finish dinner at 8:30 in the evening, I can wait until after 8:30 the next morning to eat my first meal. That adds up to at least 12 hours of "fasting."

What if I wait until 9:30, 10:30, 11:30, or even 12:30 before I eat my first meal? Waiting until 12:30 would mean that I'm giving my body a rest from the work of digestion for a full 16 hours.

I personally can tell you that I practice this second type of Intermittent Fasting regularly, and as a result feel energized and focused during and after refraining from eating for 14 or 16 hours. And as a result, I'm enjoyably hungry for a lunch meal around 12:30pm or 1:00pm.

If I desire, I can also eat a snack later in the afternoon (water first), and begin dinner by 7 or 7:30.

Intermittent Fasting is an impressive tool for weight-loss and overall health for the following reasons:

Intermittent Fasting is easy.

When you only have to prepare (or think about) two meals a day instead of three, you need less time to spend on shopping, cooking, eating, and cleaning up. (Of course, to consume the calories you need, you can enjoy healthy snacks between meals.)

Intermittent Fasting saves you money.

When you only have to prepare two meals a day instead of three, you need to purchase fewer items for your meals.

Intermittent Fasting can help improve your body's sensitivity to insulin --- which, as you read about in the last twenty-one days --- is crucial to managing weight-loss or preventing weight gain.

Intermittent Fasting promotes an increased secretion of human growth hormone (HGH), which is a key ingredient for weight-loss and muscle gain.

Intermittent Fasting can reset the imbalance of the hormones you read about --- insulin, leptin, and ghrelin --- that are influential in how hungry you are, how much you eat, and how satisfied you are after you've eaten.

Intermittent Fasting is a powerful tool because it can help reset your eating habits in general.

Refraining from eating for 12, 14, 16, or even 18 hours a day can teach your mind that you are not a slave to your appetite. Recognizing that you don't have to be a slave is very empowering. Intermittent Fasting can help you regain your sense of self-control.

Caution:

If you are someone who suffers from hypoglycemia, diabetes, an inability to regulate blood sugar, or another illness that is dependent on a regular intake of calories, please check with your doctor or health professional before experimenting with Intermittent Fasting. It can help with each of these issues, but supervision might be necessary.

Follow the advice in this guide for the kinds of foods you should be eating during the hours that you do eat! It's not a good idea to practice Intermittent Fasting when and if you're eating foods that are highly processed.

On the other hand, when you start on your first few days of Intermittent Fasting, it's possible that you'll feel grumpy or irritable. After all, you're not eating breakfast at your "regular time."

If this is the case, on the next day, delay eating breakfast one hour later than you're used to eating. Then the day after that, wait two extra hours, then three, then four, and so on. Eventually, your body will catch up with your mind and your will.

In the meantime relax, and ready yourself to begin the next exciting leg of your journey…!

Today's Goal: See how many hours you can go before eating your first meal. Remember to start the day with a glass of cool, refreshing water, and continue to drink water or teas during the hours you are refraining from eating.

Enjoy!

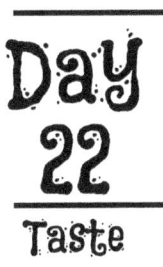

Day 22
Taste

A TASTEFUL REWARD

You've stayed with me for twenty-one days, and for that, you deserve a reward --- a reward for a job well-done.

Celebrating even small victories is therapeutic.

And completing a 21-day guide is more than a small victory.

So celebrate.

Eat a piece of chocolate!

If you choose the right kind of chocolate, you can still help yourself lose weight.

Dark chocolate --- with a content of at least 70% cacao --- is the right kind of chocolate.

A high cacao concentration in a dark chocolate bar means the following two things:

That there's less sugar in the bar (which you now know is a good thing).

That the chocolate will be less sweet (which might take some getting used to).

But what there are *more of* in a 70% dark chocolate bar are healthy fats and beneficial *antioxidant polyphenols*.

Because dark chocolate contains healthy fats, eating one or two pieces of dark chocolate (70% cacao or more) can help put your appetite in check.

Because dark chocolate contains theobromine and caffeine,

eating one or two pieces of dark chocolate (70% cacao or more) can stop you from craving other sweets.

Because of cacao's other beneficial flavanols, eating one or two pieces of dark chocolate (70% cacao or more) can help restore insulin sensitivity.

The American Journal of Clinical Nutrition published a study in March of 2005 showing how dark chocolate increased insulin sensitivity in its subjects, and from your daily journeying with me, you now understand how important being sensitive to insulin is, both for your weight and for your overall health.

Besides theobromine and caffeine, dark chocolate also contains serotonin, and serotonin cooperates with theobromine and caffeine to improve your mood…

May this celebration fill you with joy --- and leave you inspired to complete a *second* 21-day journey through this guide with me.

By the way, just say "No" to milk chocolate.

The milk added to chocolate can prevent your body from absorbing any of its beneficial antioxidants. Plus, milk chocolate is usually loaded with sugar.

And when eating chocolate, remember Goldilocks: eat just two or three square pieces.

PS: A typical dark chocolate bar weighs about 3 ounces (85 grams). Three pieces would mean eating about 14 grams, or about 1/4th of a bar.

Do you have a goal in life to be strong? If so, here's a definition to remember:

> *Real strength is breaking a chocolate bar in fourths*
> *and eating only one-fourth.*

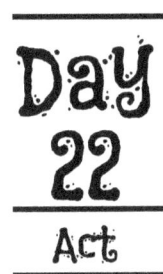

FOR THE HUNGRY TRAVELER

I've written this book to guide "hungry" travelers who have questions about how to enjoy a fit and healthy life here on this earth.

But perhaps you're a hungry traveler who has questions regarding what a person must do to enjoy a healthy life *forever*?

If you've never committed your life to knowing the Truth --- and to Jesus Christ, who is the Truth --- now would be a perfect time to begin --- in order to answer your questions.

May I suggest you buy a Bible and read it? (Why not start with the book of John?) Then locate a Bible-believing church.

You'll learn about Him, and find the answers you're seeking.

When you know the Truth, freedom in this life and the next can be yours.

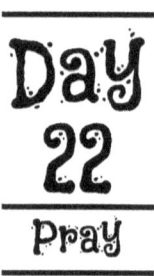

Day 22
Pray

WHERE DO I GO FROM HERE?

Thank you, God,
Thank you for taking this short journey with me,
for listening to me as I called out for help,
and for teaching me about your love and discipline.
I'm left now with quite a few things to think about,
and more than a few changes to make…
So I have one more request:
Will you continue to walk with me?
Because as I know myself, I'm thinking that there just *might* be times I'll wander off the path.
There just *might* be times that I'll slip into deep waters.
There just *might* be times that I'll need be rescued.
In my days of setbacks, will you be my support?
When I cry for help,
Will you rescue me?
And I will remain in awe that you take delight in me.

Psalm 18: 6, 16-19

In my distress I called to the Lord;
I cried to my God for help…
He reached down from on high and took hold of me;

he drew me out of deep waters.
He rescued me from my powerful enemy,
from my foes, who were too strong for me.
They confronted me in the day of my disaster,
but the Lord was my support.
He brought me out into a spacious place;
he rescued me because he delighted in me.

Psalm 119:105

Your word is a lamp for my feet,
a light on my path.

RESOURCES

DAY 1

1. "The Water in You."
Online article at: The USGS Water Science School. (Accessed Nov 2018)
https://water.usgs.gov/edu/propertyyou.html

2. Brown CM, Dulloo AG, Montani JP, "Water-induced thermogenesis reconsidered the effects of osmolality and water temperature on energy expenditure after drinking."
The Journal of Clinical Endocrinology & Metabolism. 2006 Sep; 91(9):3598-602. DOI: 10.1210/jc.2006-0407.
www.ncbi.nlm.nih.gov/pubmed/16822824

3. Stookey JD, Constant F, Popkin BM, Gardner CD, "Drinking water is associated with weight loss in overweight dieting women independent of diet and activity."
Obesity (Silver Spring). 2008 Nov; 16(11):2481-8. DOI: 10.1038/oby.2008.409.
www.ncbi.nlm.nih.gov/pubmed/18787524

4. Dennis EA, Dengo AL, Comber DL, Flack KD, Savla J, Davy KP, Davy BM, "Water consumption increases weight loss during a hypocaloric diet intervention in middle-aged and older adults."
Obesity (Silver Spring). 2010 Feb; 18(2):300-7. DOI: 10.1038/oby.2009.235.
www.ncbi.nlm.nih.gov/pubmed/?term=Dennis%20EA%5BAuthor%5D&cauthor=true&cauthor_uid=19661958

5. Parretti HM, Aveyard P, Blannin A, Clifford SJ, Coleman SJ, Roalfe A, Daley AJ, "Efficacy of water preloading before main meals as a strategy for weight loss in primary care patients with obesity: RCT."
Obesity. 2015 Sep; 23(9): 1785-1791. DOI:10.1002/oby.21167.
www.onlinelibrary.wiley.com/doi/10.1002/oby.21167/abstract

6. Boschmann M, Steiniger J, Franke G, Birkenfeld AL, Luft FC, Jordan J, "Water drinking induces thermogenesis through osmosensitive mechanisms."
Journal of Clinical Endocrinology & Metabolism. 2007 Aug; 92(8):3334-7. DOI:10.1210/jc.2006-1438.
www.ncbi.nlm.nih.gov/pubmed/17519319

7. Boschmann M, Steiniger J, Hille U, Tank J, Adams F, Sharma AM, Klaus S, Luft FC, Jordan J, "Water-induced thermogenesis."
Journal of Clinical Endocrinology & Metabolism. 2003 Dec; 88(12):6015-9. DOI: 10.1210/jc.2003-030780.
www.ncbi.nlm.nih.gov/pubmed/14671205

RESOURCES

DAY 2

1. Elliott SS, Keim NL, Stern JS, Teff K, Havel PJ, "Fructose, weight gain, and the insulin resistance syndrome."
American Journal of Clinical Lipidology. 2002 Nov; 76(5):911-922.
DOI: 10.1093/ajcn/76.5.911.
https://academic.oup.com/ajcn/article/76/5/911/4689540

2. "Is Organic Brown Rice Syrup Safe?" 2017 Mar 1.
Online Article at: drweil.com.
www.drweil.com/diet-nutrition/food-safety/is-organic-brown-rice-syrup-safe

3. Walker RW, Dumke K, Goran MI, "Fructose content in popular beverages made with and without high-fructose corn syrup."
Nutrition. 2014 Jul-Aug; Volume 30 Issues 7-8; Pages 928-935.
DOI: 10.1016/j.nut.2014.04.003.
www.sciencedirect.com/science/article/pii/S0899900714001920

4. Stanhope KL, Schwarz JM, Havel PJ, "Adverse metabolic effects of dietary fructose: results from the recent epidemiological, clinical, and mechanistic studies."
Current Opinion in Lipidology. 2013 Jun; 24(3):198-206.
DOI: 10.1097/MOL.0b013e3283613bca.
www.ncbi.nlm.nih.gov/pubmed/23594708

5. Stanhope KL et al., "Consuming fructose-sweetened, not glucose-sweetened, beverages increases visceral adiposity and lipids and decreases insulin sensitivity in overweight/obese humans."
Journal of Clinical Investigation. 2009 May; 119(5):1322-34.
DOI: 10.1172/JCI37385.
www.ncbi.nlm.nih.gov/pubmed/19381015

6. Yudkin J, *Pure, White, and Deadly* (1972, 1986, 1988, 2012, 2013)
Penguin Books, Ltd. Registered Office: 80 Strand, London WC2R 0RI, England
British nutritionist John Yudkin presents decades of research pointing at dietary sugar — rather than fat — as the underlying factor in diabetes and obesity.

7. Mercola J, "Best Foods for Boosting Brain Power." 2016 Sep 29.
Online Article at: articles.mercola.com
www.articles.mercola.com/sites/articles/archive/2016/09/29/foods-improve-brain-health.aspx

8. Mercola J, "Diet Soda Makers Sued Over Deceptive, False and Misleading Advertising." 2017 Oct 31. Online Article at: articles.mercola.com.
www.articles.mercola.com/sites/articles/archive/2017/10/31/soda-makers-false-advertising.aspx

9. Mercola J, "New Study Shows Artificial Sweeteners Can Lead to Diabetes." 2017 Oct 3. On-line Article at: articles.mercola.com.

www.articles.mercola.com/sites/articles/archive/2017/10/03/artificial-sweeteners-lead-to-diabetes.aspx

10. Mercola J, *Sweet Deception: Why Splenda, NutraSweet, and the FDA May Be Hazardous to Your Health* (2006) Thomas Nelson Publishing: Nashville, TN

11. Blaylock RL, *Excitoxins: The Taste that Kills* (1994) Health Press: P.O. Box 1388, Santa Fe, NM

12. Thibodeau GA, Patton KT, *Anatomy & Physiology, Sixth Edition* (2007) Mosby Elsevier: St. Louis, MO

13. "Coke Shouldn't Bother Rehabilitating Aspartame's Image, Says CSPI." 2013 Aug 14. Online Article at: Center For Science in the Public Interest: CSPInet.org www.cspinet.org/new/201308141.html

14. Bellisle F, Drewnowski A, "Intense sweeteners, energy intake and the control of body weight."
European Journal of Clinical Nutrition. 2007; 61:691-700.
DOI: 10.1038/sj.ejcn.1602649.
www.ncbi.nlm.nih.gov/pubmed/17299484

15. de MatosFeijó F, et al., "Saccharin and aspartame, compared with sucrose, induce greater weight gain in adult Wistar rats, at similar total caloric intake levels."
Appetite. 2012 Jan 1; Volume 60, Pages 203-207.
DOI:10.1016/j.appet.2012.10.009.
www.sciencedirect.com/science/article/pii/S0195666312004138

16. Yang Q,, "Gain weight by 'going diet?' Artificial sweeteners and the neurobiology of sugar cravings."
Yale Journal of Biology and Medicine. 2010 Jun; 83(2): 101–108. PMID: 20589192.
www.ncbi.nlm.nih.gov/pmc/articles/PMC2892765/

17. Anton SD, Martin CK, Han H, Coulon S, Cefalu WT, Geiselman P, Williamson DA, "Effects of stevia, aspartame, and sucrose on food intake, satiety, and postprandial glucose and insulin levels."
Appetite. 2010 Aug; 55(1): 37-43. DOI: 10.1016/j.appet.2010.03.009.
www.ncbi.nlm.nih.gov/pubmed/20303371

18. Hsieh MH, Chan P, Sue YM, Liu JC, Liang TH, Huang TY, Tomlinson B, Chow MS, Kao MS, Kao PF, Chen YJ, "Efficacy and tolerability of oral stevioside in patients with mild essential hypertension: a two-year, randomized, placebo-controlled study."
Clinical Therapy. 2003 Nov; 25(11):2797-808. PMID: 14693305.
www.ncbi.nlm.nih.gov/pubmed/14693305

19. Casselbury K, "Is Carbonated Water Bad for You?" 2017 Oct.
Online Article at: livestrong.com.
www.livestrong.com/article/156879-health-effects-of-carbonated-water/#sthash.0aj10IUT.dpuf

DAY 3

20. Tucker KL et al., "Colas, but not other carbonated beverages, are associated with low bone mineral density in older women: The Framingham Osteoporosis Study."
American Journal of Clinical Nutrition. 2006 Oct;84(4):936-42.
DOI: 10.1093/ajcn/84.4.936.
https://academic.oup.com/ajcn/article/84/4/936/4632980

DAY 3

1. Fushimi T1, Suruga K, Oshima Y, Fukiharu M, Tsukamoto Y, Goda T, "Dietary acetic acid reduces serum cholesterol and triacylglycerols in rats fed a cholesterol-rich diet."
British Journal of Nutrition. 2006 May; 95(5):916-24. PMID: 16611381.
www.ncbi.nlm.nih.gov/pubmed/16611381

2. Johnston CS, Kim CM, Buller AJ, "Vinegar Improves Insulin Sensitivity to a High-Carbohydrate Meal in Subjects With Insulin Resistance or Type 2 Diabetes."
Diabetes Care. 2004 Jan; 27(1): 281-282. DOI:10.2337/diacare.27.1.281.
care.diabetesjournals.org/content/27/1/281.full

3. Ostman E1, Granfeldt Y, Persson L, Björck I, "Vinegar supplementation lowers glucose and insulin responses and increases satiety after a bread meal in healthy subjects."
European Journal of Clinical Nutrition. 2005 Sep; 59(9):983-8.
DOI:10.1038/sj.ejcn.1602197.
www.ncbi.nlm.nih.gov/pubmed/16015276

4. Kondo T, Kishi M, Fushimi T, Ugajin S, Kaga T, "Vinegar intake reduces body weight, body fat mass, and serum triglyceride levels in obese Japanese subjects."
Bioscience, Biotechnology, and Biochemistry. 2009 Aug; 73(8):1837-43.
PMID: 19661687.
www.ncbi.nlm.nih.gov/pubmed/19661687

5. Corleone J, "Can Apple Cider Vinegar Help Digestion?" (Last Updated: 2017 Oct 03).
Online Article at: livestrong.com
www.livestrong.com/article/530301-can-apple-cider-vinegar-help-digestion

DAY 4

1. Acheson KJ, Gremaud G, Meirim I, Montigon F, Krebs Y, Fay LB, Gay L-J, Schneiter P, Schindler C, and Tappy L, "Metabolic effects of caffeine in humans: lipid oxidation or futile cycling?"
American Journal of Clinical Nutrition. 2004 Jan; 79 (1): 40-6.
DOI: 10.1093/ajcn/79.1.40.
https://www.ncbi.nlm.nih.gov/pubmed/14684395

2. Doherty M, Smith PM, "Effects of caffeine ingestion on rating of perceived exertion during and after exercise: a meta-analysis."
Scandinavian Journal of Medicine & Science in Sports. 2005 Mar 18; Volume 15, Issue 2. DOI: 10.1111/j.1600-0838.2005.00445.x.
www.onlinelibrary.wiley.com/doi/10.1111/j.1600-0838.2005.00445.x/abstract

3. Koithan M, Niemeyer K, "Using Herbal Remedies to Maintain Optimal Weight."
The Journal for Nurse Practitioners. 2010 Feb; 6(2): 153–154.
DOI: 10:1016/j.nurpra.2009.12.005.
https://www.npjournal.org/article/S1555-4155(09)00685-0/fulltext

4. Dulloo AG, Duret C, Rohrer D, Girardier L, Mensi N, Fathi M, Chantre P, Vandermander J, "Efficacy of a green tea extract rich in catechin polyphenols and caffeine in increasing 24-h energy expenditure and fat oxidation in humans."
American Journal of Clinical Nutrition. 1999 Dec; 70(6):1040-5.
DOI: 10.1093/ajcn/70.6.1040.
www.ncbi.nlm.nih.gov/pubmed/10584049

5. Maki KC et al., "Green Tea Catechin Consumption Enhances Exercise-Induced Abdominal Fat Loss in Overweight and Obese Adults."
The Journal of Nutrition. 2009 Feb; 139(2):264-70. DOI: 10.3945/jn.108.098293.
https://www.ncbi.nlm.nih.gov/pubmed/19074207

6. Carter BE, Drewnowski A, "Beverages containing soluble fiber, caffeine, and green tea catechins suppress hunger and lead to less energy consumption at the next meal."
Appetite. 2012 Dec; 59(3):755-61. DOI: 10.1016/j.appet.2012.08.015.
www.ncbi.nlm.nih.gov/pubmed/22922604

7. Riegsecker S, Wiczynski D, Kaplan MJ, Ahmed S, "Potential benefits of green tea polyphenol EGCG in the prevention and treatment of vascular inflammation in rheumatoid arthritis."
Life Science. 2013 Sep 3; 93(8):307-12. DOI: 10.1016/j.lfs.2013.07.006
www.ncbi.nlm.nih.gov/pubmed/23871988

8. Newsome BJ, Petriello MC, Han SG, Murphy MO, Eske KE, Sunkara M, Morris AJ, Hennig B, "Green tea diet decreases PCB 126-induced oxidative stress in mice by up-regulating antioxidant enzymes."
Journal of Nutritional Biochemistry. 2014 Feb; 25(2):126-35.
DOI: 10.1016/j.jnutbio.2013.10.003.
www.ncbi.nlm.nih.gov/pubmed/24378064

9. Betts JW, Wareham DW, Haswell SJ, Kelly SM, "Antifungal synergy of theaflavin and epicatechin combinations against Candida albicans."
Journal of Microbiology and Biotechnology. 2013 Sep 28; 23(9):1322-6.
PMID: 23711519.
https://www.ncbi.nlm.nih.gov/pubmed/23711519

DAY 5

1. Stein R, "Research Links Obesity to Mix of Bacteria in Digestive Tract." *Washington Post.* 2006 Dec 12.
www.washingtonpost.com/wp-dyn/content/article/2006/12/20/AR2006122001271.html

2. Williams D, "9 Ways Good Gut Bacteria Support Your Overall Health (That Have Nothing to Do With Digestion)." (Accessed Dec 2018)
Online Article at: drdavidwilliams.com.
www.drdavidwilliams.com/9-ways-good-gut-bacteria-support-your-overall-health

3. Ridaura V et al., "Gut Microbiota from Twins Discordant for Obesity Modulate Metabolism in Mice."
Science. 2013 Sept 06; Vol 341, Issue 6150, 1241212.
DOI: 10.1126/science.1241214.
science.sciencemag.org/content/341/6150/1241214

4. Wallis C, "How Gut Bacteria Help Make Us Fat and Thin."
Scientific American. 2014 Jun 1.
www.scientificamerican.com/article/how-gut-bacteria-help-make-us-fat-and-thin

5. Sanchez M. et al, "Effect of Lactobacillus rhamnosus CGMCC1.3724 supplementation on weight loss and maintenance in obese men and women."
British Journal of Nutrition. 2014 April 28; Volume 111, Issue 8, pp. 1507-1519.
DOI: 10.1017/S0007114513003875.
https://www.cambridge.org/core/journals/british-journal-of-nutrition/article/effect-of-lactobacillus-rhamnosus-cgmcc13724-supplementation-on-weight-loss-and-maintenance-in-obese-men-and-women/7C9810D79528C4ADC77A22EE45F9CA8E

6. Tremblay A et al., "Certain probiotics could help women lose weight."
Source: Jean-François Huppé, Faculty of Medicine, Université Laval. 28 January 2018. Online Article at: Université Laval.
www.ulaval.ca/en/about-us/media-center/press-releases/details/article/certain-probiotics-could-help-women-lose-weight.html

7. Weed S, "News on Healthy Weight -- Cultures in Yogurt Help Women Stay Shapely."
Online Article at: Wise Woman Tradition (Accessed July 2018).
www.wisewomantradition.com/wisewomanweb/2014/04/cultures-in-yogurt-help-women-stay-shapely.html

DAY 6

1. Dean C, *The Magnesium Miracle* (2007) Ballantine Books: New York, NY

2. Durlach J, Pagès N, Bac P, Bara M, Guiet-Bara A, "Biorhythms and possible

central regulation of magnesium status, phototherapy, darkness therapy and chronopathological forms of magnesium depletion."
Magnesium Research. 2002 Mar; 15(1-2):49-66. PMID:12030424
www.ncbi.nlm.nih.gov/pubmed/12030424

3. Rosedale R, "Leptin—Its Essential Role in Health, Disease, and Aging." Online Article at: drrosedale.com (Accessed July 2018).
drrosedale.com/resources/pdf/Leptin%20and%20its%20essential%20role%20in%20health%20disease%20and%20aging.pdf

4. Otero et al., "Towards a pro-inflammatory and immunomodulatory emerging role of leptin."
Rheumatology (Oxford). 2006 Aug; 45:944–50.
DOI: 10.1093/rheumatology/kel157.
www.ncbi.nlm.nih.gov/pubmed/16720637

5. Ahima RS, Prabakaran D, Mantzoros C, Qu D, Lowell B, Maratos-Flier E, Flier JS, "Role of leptin in the neuroendocrine response to fasting."
Nature. 1996 Jul 18; 382(6588):250-2. DOI: 10.1038/382250a0.
www.ncbi.nlm.nih.gov/pubmed/8717038

6. Considine RV, Sinha MK, Heiman ML, Kriauciunas A, Stephens TW, Nyce MR, Ohannesian JP, Marco CC, McKee, LJ, Bauer, TL, et al., "Serum immunoreactive-leptin concentrations in normal-weight and obese humans."
New England Journal of Medicine. 1996 Feb 1; 334(5): 292–5.
DOI: 10.1056/NEJM199602013340503.
www.ncbi.nlm.nih.gov/pubmed/8532024

7. Nielsen F H, Johnson LK, Zeng H, "Magnesium supplementation improves indicators of low magnesium status and inflammatory stress in adults older than 51 years with poor quality sleep."
Magnesium Research. 2010 Dec; 23.4 (4):158-168. DOI: 10.1684/mrh.2010.0220.
https://www.researchgate.net/publication/49722621_Magnesium_supplementation_improves_indicators_of_low_magnesium_status_and_inflammatory_stress_in_adults_older_than_51_years_with_poor_quality_sleep

8. Held K, Antonijevic IA, Künzel H, et al., "Oral Mg(2+) supplementation reverses age-related neuroendocrine and sleep EEG changes in humans."
Pharmacopsychiatry. 2002 Jul; 35(4):135-43. DOI: 10.1055/s-2002-33195
www.ncbi.nlm.nih.gov/pubmed/12163983

9. Abbasi B, Kimiagar M, Sadeghniiat K, et al., "The effect of magnesium supplementation on primary insomnia in elderly: A double-blind placebo-controlled clinical trial."
International Journal of Research in Medical Sciences. 2012 Dec; 17(12):1161-9.
PMID: 23853635.
www.ncbi.nlm.nih.gov/pubmed/23853635

10. Durlach J, Pagès N, Bac P, Bara M, Guiet-Bara A. "Biorhythms and possible central regulation of magnesium status, phototherapy, darkness therapy and

DAY 7

chronopathological forms of magnesium depletion."
Magnesium Research. 2002 Mar; 15(1-2):49-66. PMID:12030424.
www.ncbi.nlm.nih.gov/pubmed/12030424

11. Hyman M, "Magnesium: Meet the Most Powerful Relaxation Mineral Available."
Online Article at: Mark Hyman, MD Blog (May 2010).
www.drhyman.com/blog/2010/05/20/magnesium-the-most-powerful-relaxation-mineral-available

12. Song Y, Dai Q., He K, "Magnesium Intake, Insulin Resistance, and Type 2 Diabetes."
North American Journal of Medicine and Science. 2013 Jan; Vol 6 No 1.
DOI: 10.7156/najms.2013.0601009.
www.zoelho.com/ZoelhoFR/Publish/Magn_diabetes.pdf

13. Dong JY, Xun P, He K, Qin LQ, "Magnesium intake and risk of type 2 diabetes: meta-analysis of prospective cohort studies."
Diabetes Care. 2011 Sep; 34(9):2116-22. DOI: 10.2337/dc11-0518.
www.ncbi.nlm.nih.gov/pubmed/21868780

14. Larsson SC, Wolk A, "Magnesium intake and risk of type 2 diabetes: a meta-analysis."
Journal of Internal Medicine. 2007 Aug; 262(2)208-14.
DOI: 10.1111/j.1365-2796.2007.01840.x.
www.ncbi.nlm.nih.gov/pubmed/17645588

15. Rodriguez-Moran M, Simental Mendia LE, Zambrano Galván G, Guerrero-Romero F, "The role of magnesium in type 2 diabetes: a brief based-clinical review."
Magnesium Research. 2011 Dec; 24(4)156-62. DOI: 10.1684/mrh.2011.0299.
www.ncbi.nlm.nih.gov/pubmed/22198525

16. Singh RB, Beegom R, Rastogi Ss, Gaoli A, Shoumin Z, "Association of low plasma concentrations of antioxidant vitamins, magnesium and zinc with high body fat percent measured by bioelectrical impedance analysis in Indian men."
*Magnesium Research.*1998 Mar; 11(1):3-10. PMID: 9595544.
https://www.ncbi.nlm.nih.gov/pubmed/9595544

17. Aikawa JK, *Magnesium: Its Biological Significance* (1981) CRC Press: Boca Raton, FL

DAY 7

1. Mercola J, "How High-Fructose Corn Syrup Damages Your Body." 2007 Jul 24. Online Article at: mercola.com.
https://articles.mercola.com/sites/articles/archive/2007/07/10/how-high-fructose-corn-syrup-damages-your-body.aspx

2. Pandey KB, Rizvi SI, "Plant polyphenols as dietary antioxidants in human

health and disease."
Oxidative Medicine and Cellular Longevity. 2009 Nov-Dec; 2(5): 270–278.
DOI: 10.4161/oxim.2.5.9498.
http://www.ncbi.nlm.nih.gov/pmc/articles/PMC2835915

3. Fernández de Simon B, Perez-Ilzarbe J, Hernandez T, Gomez-Cordoves C, Estrella I, "Importance of phenolic compounds for the characterization of fruit juices."
Journal of Agricultural and Food Chemistry. 1992 Sep; 40:1531–1535.
DOI: 10.1021/jf00021a012.
https://pubs.acs.org/doi/abs/10.1021/jf00021a012

4. Julie Upton, MS RD "Does Fiber Help You Lose Weight, and Other Burning Diet Questions." 2008 Apr 25.
Online Article at: Health.com www.health.com/type-2-diabetes/does-fiber-help-you-lose-weight

5. Ferrari N, "Making one change --- getting more fiber --- can help with weight loss." (Updated April 9, 2015).
Online Article at: Harvard Health Blog: health.harvard.edu.
www.health.harvard.edu/blog/making-one-change-getting-fiber-can-help-weight-loss-201502177721

6. Jobgen W, Meininger CJ, Jobgen SC, Li P, Lee MJ, Smith SB, Spencer TE, Fried SK, Wu G, "Dietary L-arginine supplementation reduces white fat gain and enhances skeletal muscle and brown fat masses in diet-induced obese rats."
Journal of Nutrition. 2009 Feb; 139(2): 230-7. DOI: 10.3945/jn.108.096362.
www.ncbi.nlm.nih.gov/pubmed/19106310

7. Johnston CS, Corte C, Swan PD, "Marginal vitamin C status is associated with reduced fat oxidation during submaximal exercise in young adults."
Nutrition & Metabolism (Lond). 2006 Aug 31; 3:35.
DOI: 10.1186/1743-7075-3-35.
www.ncbi.nlm.nih.gov/pubmed/16945143?dopt=Abstract

DAY 8

1. Abelow BJ, Holford TR, Insogna KL, "Cross-cultural association between dietary animal protein and hip fracture: a hypothesis."
Calcified Tissue International. 1992 Jan; 50(1):14-8. PMID: 1739864.
www.ncbi.nlm.nih.gov/pubmed/1739864

2. Feskanich D, Willett WC, Stampfer MJ, Colditz GA, "Milk, dietary calcium, and bone fractures in women: a 12-year prospective study."
American Journal of Public Health. 1997 Jun; 87(6):992-7. PMID: 9224182.
www.ncbi.nlm.nih.gov/pubmed/9224182

3. "Feeling Great With Cruciferous Vegetables."
Online Article at: whfoods.org (Accessed July 2018).

DAY 9

www.whfoods.com/genpage.php?tname=btnews&dbid=125

4. Slavin JL, Ph.D., "Dietary fiber and body weight."
Nutrition. 2005 Mar; Volume 21, Issue 3, Pages 411-418.
Review article at: sciencedirect.com.
www.sciencedirect.com/science/article/pii/S0899900704003041

5. Stenblom EL, Egecioglu E, Landin-Olsson M, Erlanson-Albertsson C, "Consumption of thylakoid-rich spinach extract reduces hunger, increases satiety and reduces cravings for palatable food in overweight women."
Appetite. 2015 Aug; 91:209-19. DOI: 10.1016/j.appet.2015.04.051.
www.ncbi.nlm.nih.gov/pubmed/25895695

6. "Reducing hunger, weight and sugar cravings with green gold." 2015 Oct 22.
Online Article at: Nutraceutical Business Review.
www.nutraceuticalbusinessreview.com/technical/article_page/Reducing_hunger_weight_and_sugar_cravings_with_green_gold/112873

7. Akesson A, "Gary Taubes on What He Eats for Breakfast and Why America is Fat." 2017 April.
Online Article at: dietdoctor.com.
www.dietdoctor.com/gary-taubes-eats-breakfast-america-fat

DAY 9

1. Marx W, Kiss N, Isenring L, "Is ginger beneficial for nausea and vomiting? An update of the literature."
Current Opinion in Supportive and Palliative Care. 2015 Jun; 9(2):189-95.
DOI: 10.1097/SPC.0000000000000135.
www.ncbi.nlm.nih.gov/pubmed/25872115

2. Ernst E, Pittler MH, "Efficacy of ginger for nausea and vomiting: a systematic review of randomized clinical trials."
British Journal Anaesthesia. 2000 Mar; 84(3):367-71. PMID: 10793599.
www.ncbi.nlm.nih.gov/pubmed/10793599

3. Viljoen E, Visser J, Koen N, Musekiwa A, "A systematic review and meta-analysis of the effect and safety of ginger in the treatment of pregnancy-associated nausea and vomiting."
Nutrition Journal. 2014 Mar 19; 13:20. DOI: 10.1186/1475-2891-13-20.
www.ncbi.nlm.nih.gov/pmc/articles/PMC3995184

4. Mansour MS, Ni YM, Roberts AL, Kelleman M, Roychoudhury A, St-Onge MP, "Ginger consumption enhances the thermic effect of food and promotes feelings of satiety without affecting metabolic and hormonal parameters in overweight men: a pilot study."
Metabolism. 2012 Oct; 61(10):1346-52. DOI: 10.1016/j.metabol.2012.03.016.
www.ncbi.nlm.nih.gov/pubmed/22538118

5. Khandouzi N, Shidfar F, Rajab A, Rahideh T, Hosseini P, Mir Taheri M, "The

effects of ginger on fasting blood sugar, hemoglobin a1c, apolipoprotein B, apolipoprotein a-l and malondialdehyde in type 2 diabetic patients."
Iranian Journal of Pharmaceutical Research. 2015 Winter; 14(1):131-40. PMID: 25561919.
www.ncbi.nlm.nih.gov/pubmed/25561919

6. Altman RD, Marcussen KC, "Effects of a ginger extract on knee pain in patients with osteoarthritis."
Arthritis & Rheumatology. 2001 Nov; 44(11):2531-8. PMID: 11710709.
www.ncbi.nlm.nih.gov/pubmed/11710709

7. Black CD, Herring MP, Hurley DJ, O'Connor PJ, "Ginger (Zingiber officinale) reduces muscle pain caused by eccentric exercise."
The Journal of Pain. 2010 Sep; 11(9):894-903. DOI: 10.1016/j.jpain.2009.12.013.
www.ncbi.nlm.nih.gov/pubmed/20418184

DAY 10

1. Elkayam A, Mirelman D, Peleg E, Wilchek M, Miron T, Rabinkov A, Oron-Herman M, Rosenthal T, "The effects of allicin on weight in fructose-induced hyperinsulinemic, hyperlipidemic, hypertensive rats."
American Journal of Hypertension. 2003 Dec; Volume 16, Issue 12, Pages 1053-1056. DOI: 10.1016/j.amjhyper.2003.07.011.
www.ajh.oxfordjournals.org/content/16/12/1053.short

2. Seo DY, Lee SR, Kim HK, Baek YH, Kwak YS, Ko TH, Kim N, Rhee BD, Ko KS, Park BJ, Han J, "Independent Beneficial Effects of Aged Garlic Extract Intake with Regular Exercise on Cardiovascular Risk in Postmenopausal Women."
Nutrition Research and Practice. 2012 June; 6(3): 226- 231.
DOI: 10.4162/nrp.2012.6.3.226.
www.ncbi.nlm.nih.gov/pmc/articles/PMC3395788

3. Chapman J, "Why garlic can help you lose weight."
Online Article at: dailymail.com (Accessed July 2018).
www.dailymail.co.uk/health/article-87815/Why-garlic-help-lose-weight.html

DAY 11

1. Sears A, "The Awful Truth About Turmeric."
Online Article at: Wellness Research and Consulting Inc. (Accessed Dec 2018).
www.primalforce.net/landingp/curcumin-turmeric-delivers-over-619-known-health-benefits/?futm_campaign=jvout_inhr_curcumin_awful_truth_turmeric_20161015_let&futm_source=inhr&futm_medium=-jvout

2. "What's New and Beneficial About Turmeric."
Online Article at: whfoods.com (Accessed Oct 2018).
www.whfoods.com/genpage.php?tname=foodspice&dbid=78

3. Nagabhushan M, Bhide SV, "Curcumin as an inhibitor of cancer."
Journal of the American College of Nutrition. 1992 Apr;11(2):192-8. 1992.
PMID:1578097.
https://www.ncbi.nlm.nih.gov/pubmed/1578097

4. Yu Y, Hu SK, Yan H; "The study of insulin resistance and leptin resistance on the model of simplicity obesity rats by curcumin."
Zhongjua Yu Fang Yi Xue Za Ahi. 2008 Nov;42(11): 818-22.
PMID: 19176142.
http://www.ncbi.nlm.nih.gov/pubmed/19176142

5. "Turmeric Extract Suppresses Fat Tissue Growth in Rodent Models."
Online at: Tufts Now. 2009 May 18.
https://now.tufts.edu/news-releases/turmeric-extract-suppresses-fat-tissue-growth

6. Di Pierro F, Bressan A, Ranaldi D, Rapacioli G, Giacomelli L, Bertuccioli A, "Potential role of bioavailable curcumin in weight loss and omental adipose tissue decrease: preliminary data of a randomized, controlled trial in overweight people with metabolic syndrome. Preliminary study."
European Review for Medical and Pharmacological Sciences. 2015 Nov; 19(21):4195-202. PMID: 26592847.
www.ncbi.nlm.nih.gov/pubmed/26592847

7. Cespedes A, "Turmeric & Weight Loss."
Online Article at: livestrong.com. 2017 Jul 18.
www.livestrong.com/article/247386-turmeric-weight-loss/#sthash.oELmOnnk.dpuf

DAY 12

1. Janssens PLHR, Hursel R, Martens EAP, Westerterp-Plantenga MS, "Acute Effects of Capsaicin on Energy Expenditure and Fat Oxidation in Negative Energy Balance."
PLoS One. 2013 Jul; 8(7): e67786. DOI: 10.1371/journal.pone.0067786.
www.ncbi.nlm.nih.gov/pubmed/23844093

2. Hursel R, Westerterp-Plantenga MS, "Thermogenic ingredients and body weight regulation."
International Journal of Obesity (Lond). 2010 Apr; 34(4):659-6.
DOI: 10.1038/ijo.2009.299.
www.ncbi.nlm.nih.gov/pubmed/20142827

3. Neubert AP, "Study: Reasonable quantities of red pepper may help curb appetite."
Online Article at: Purdue University News Service 2011 Apr 25.
www.purdue.edu/newsroom/research/2011/110425MattesPepper.html

4. Ludy MJ, Mattes RD, "The effects of hedonically acceptable red pepper doses on thermogenesis and appetite."
Physiology & Behavior. 2011 Mar 1; 102(3-4):251-8.

DOI: 10.1016/j.physbeh.2010.11.018.
www.ncbi.nlm.nih.gov/pubmed/21093467

5. Whiting S, Derbyshire E, Tiwari BK, "Capsaicinoids and capsinoids. A potential role for weight management? A systematic review of the evidence." *Appetite.* 2012 Oct;59(2):341-8. DOI: 10.1016/j.appet.2012.05.015.
www.ncbi.nlm.nih.gov/pubmed/22634197

6. Joo JI, Kim DH, Choi JW, Yun JW, "Proteomic analysis for antiobesity potential of capsaicin on white adipose tissue in rats fed with a high fat diet." *Journal of Proteome Research.* 2010 Jun 4; 9(6):2977-87. DOI: 10.1021/pr901175w.
www.ncbi.nlm.nih.gov/pubmed/20359164

DAY 13

1. Castro RM, "Is it true that cinnamon can lower blood sugar in people who have diabetes?"
Online Article at: mayoclinic.org (Accessed Nov 2018).
www.mayoclinic.org/diseases-conditions/diabetes/expert-answers/diabetes/faq-20058472

2. Kirkham S, Akilen R, Sharma S, Tsiami A, "The potential of cinnamon to reduce blood glucose levels in patients with type 2 diabetes and insulin resistance."
Diabetes, Obesity and Metabolism. 2009 Nov 10; Volume 11, Issue 12.
DOI: 10.1111/j.1463-1326.2009.01094.x. (Accessed at: wileyonlinelibrary.com)
www.onlinelibrary.wiley.com/doi/10.1111/j.1463-1326.2009.01094.x

3. "Cinnamon Benefits."
Online Article at: herbwisdom.com (Accessed July 2018).
www.herbwisdom.com/herb-cinnamon.html

4. Qin B, Panickar KS, Anderson RA, "Cinnamon: Potential Role in the Prevention of Insulin Resistance, Metabolic Syndrome, and Type 2 Diabetes."
Journal of Diabetes Science and Technology. 2010 May; 4(3): 685-693.
DOI: 10.1177/193229681000400324.
www.ncbi.nlm.nih.gov/pmc/articles/PMC2901047

5. Hlebowicz J, Darwiche G, Bjorgell O, Almér LO, "Effect of cinnamon on postprandial blood glucose, gastric emptying, and satiety in healthy subjects."
American Journal of Clinical Nutrition. 2007 June; 85(6): 1552-6.
DOI: 10.1093/ajcn/85.6.1552.
www.ncbi.nlm.nih.gov/pubmed/17556692

6. Graedon J, "Cinnamon Offers Health Benefits but Also Carries Serious Risks."
Online Article at: The People's Pharmacy 2018 Dec 30.
www.peoplespharmacy.com/2013/12/30/cinnamon-offers-health-benefits-but-also-carries-serious-risks

DAY 14

1. Simopoulos AP, "Essential fatty acids in health and chronic disease."
American Journal of Clinical Nutrition. 1999 Sep; 70(3 Suppl):560S-569S.
DOI: 10.1093/ajcn/70.3.560s.
www.ncbi.nlm.nih.gov/pubmed/10479232

2. Adolphe JL, Whiting SJ, Juurlink BH, Thorpe LU, Alcorn J, "Health effects with consumption of the flax lignan secoisolariciresinol diglucoside."
British Journal of Nutrition. 2010 April 14; Volume 103 , pp. 929-938.
DOI: 10.1017/S0007114509992753.
www.cambridge.org/core/journals/british-journal-of-nutrition/article/health-effects-with-consumption-of-the-flax-lignan-secoisolariciresinol-diglucoside/5D2166DC186CD6C723DF07907683CF83

3. Mercola J, "The Health Benefits of Fiber."
Online Article at: mercola.com 2013 Nov 25.
www.articles.mercola.com/sites/articles/archive/2013/11/25/9-fiber-health-benefits.aspx

4. Mayo Clinic Staff, "Dietary fiber: Essential for a healthy diet."
Online Article at: Healthy Lifestyle: Nutrition and healthy eating/Mayo Clinic.org (Accessed July 2018).
www.mayoclinic.org/healthy-lifestyle/nutrition-and-healthy-eating/in-depth/fiber/art-20043983

5. Mercola J, "What is Flaxseed Good For?"
Online Article at: mercola.com 2015 Sep 22.
www.foodfacts.mercola.com/flaxseed.html

6. Mercola J, "How to Know When Flax Is Rancid."
Online Article at: mercola.com 2017 Feb 25.
www.articles.mercola.com/sites/articles/archive/2017/02/25/how-to-know-when-flaxseed-is-rancid.aspx

DAY 15

1. Prior A, Davidson F, Salmond CE, Czochanska Z, "Cholesterol, coconuts, and diet on Polynesian atolls: a natural experiment: the Pukapuka and Tokelau island studies."
American Journal of Clinical Nutrition. 1981 Aug; 34(8):1552-61.
DOI: 10.1093/ajcn/34.8.1552.
https://www.ncbi.nlm.nih.gov/pubmed/7270479

2. Evans M, Sinclair RC, Fusimalohi C, Liava'a V, "Globalization, diet, and health: an example from Tonga."
Online Paper: Special Theme: "Globalization."
www.ncbi.nlm.nih.gov/pmc/articles/PMC2566641/pdf/11584734.pdf

3. Fife B, *Eat Fat Look Thin: A Safe and Natural Way to Lose Weight Permanently* (2005) Piccadilly Books: Ltd. Colorado Springs, CO

4. Taubes G, "What If It's All Been a Big Fat Lie?"
The New York Times Magazine 2002 July 7.
www.nytimes.com/2002/07/07/magazine/what-if-it-s-all-been-a-big-fat-lie.html

5. Brown, MJ, Ferruzzi MG, Nguyen ML, Cooper DA, Eldridge AL, Schwartz SJ, White WS, "Carotenoid bioavailability is higher from salads ingested with full-fat than with fat-reduced salad dressings as measured with electrochemical detection."
American Journal of Clinical Nutrition. 2004 Aug; vol 80: pp 396-403.
DOI: 10.1093/ajcn/80.2.396.
www.academic.oup.com/ajcn/article/80/2/396/4690323

6. Hata T, Guerrero-Juarez CF, Ramos P, Plikus MV, Bapat SP, "Fat isn't all bad: Skin adipocytes help protect against infections."
Online Article at: eurekalert.org/AAAS (The Global Source for Science News). Article from: University of California-San Diego 2015 Jan.
https://www.eurekalert.org/pub_releases/2015-01/uoc--fia122914.php

7. Zhang L, Guerrero-Juarez CF, Hata Tissa, Bapat SP, Ramos R, Plikus MV, Gallo RL, "Dermal adipocytes protect against invasive Staphylococcus aureus skin infection."
Science. 2015 Jan 2; 347(6217):67-71. DOI: 1126/science. 1260972.
https://www.ncbi.nlm.nih.gov/pubmed/25554785

8. Mercola J, "Fat Beneath Skin May Ward Off Infections."
Online Article at: mercola.com 2015 Jan 17.
www.articles.mercola.com/sites/articles/archive/2015/01/17/skin-fat-may-ward-off-infections.aspx

9. Teicholz N, *The Big Fat Surprise* (2014) Simon & Schuster: New York, NY
(*In a 1952 study performed at the Institute for Metabolic Research in Oakland, California researchers first discovered that total cholesterol levels could be lowered if subjects replaced animal fats --- or saturated fats --- with vegetable oils [pg. 26]. ...Ancel Keys believed that the total amount of dietary fat better determined heart disease risk than the type of fat...and small experiments Keys himself conducted showed that lower-fat diets performed slightly better in lowering cholesterol. Keys promoted the results as if there were already little room for doubt [pg. 27]. [Nevertheless] a large number of experiments have since confirmed that restricting fat does nothing to slim people down {quite the reverse, actually}...[pg. 29]. Nina Teicholz, The Big Fat Surprise.*)

10. Ravnskov U et al., "Lack of an association or an inverse association between low-density-lipoprotein cholesterol and mortality in the elderly; a systematic review."
British Medical Journal Open. 2016 Jun 12; 6(6):e010401.
DOI: 10.1136/bmjopen-2015-010401.
https://www.ncbi.nlm.nih.gov/pubmed/27292972

11. Hayek T, Ito Y, Azrolan N, Verdery RB, Aalto-Setälä, Walsh A, Breslow JL, "Dietary fat increases high density lipoprotein (HDL) levels both by increasing the transport rates and decreasing the fractional catabolic rates of HDL cholesterol ester and apolipoprotein (Apo) A-l. Presentation of a new animal model and mechanistic studies in human Apo A-I transgenic and control mice."
Journal of Clinical Investigation. 1993 Apr; 91(4): 1665-1671.
DOI: 10.1172/JCI116375.
www.ncbi.nlm.nih.gov/pmc/articles/PMC288145

12. Abargouei AS, Janghorbani M, Salehi-Marzijarani M, Esmaillzadeh A, "Effect of dairy consumption on weight and body composition in adults: a systematic review and meta-analysis of randomized controlled clinical trials."
International Journal of Obesity (Lond): 2012 Dec; 36(12):1485-93
DOI: 10.1038/ijo.2011.269.
www.ncbi.nlm.nih.gov/pubmed/22249225

13. Stubbs RJ, Harbron CG, "Covert manipulation of the ratio of medium- to long-chain triglycerides in isoenergetically dense diets: effect on food intake in ad libitum feeding men."
International Journal of Obesity and Related Metabolic Disorders. 1996 May; 20(5):435-44. PMID: 8696422.
www.ncbi.nlm.nih.gov/pubmed/8696422

14. Dulloo AG, Fathi M, Mensi N, Girardier L, "Twenty-four-hour energy expenditure and urinary catecholamines of humans consuming low-to-moderate amounts of medium-chain triglycerides: a dose-response study in a human respiratory chamber."
European Journal of Clinical Nutrition. 1996 Mar; 50(3):152-8. PMID: 8654328.
www.ncbi.nlm.nih.gov/pubmed/8654328

15. Van Wymelbeke V, Himaya A, Louis-Sylvestre J, Fantino M, "Influence of medium-chain and long-chain triacylglycerols on the control of food intake in men."
American Journal of Clinical Nutrition. 1998 Aug; 68(2):226-34.
DOI: 10.1093/ajcn/68.2.226.
www.ncbi.nlm.nih.gov/pubmed/9701177

16. St-Onge MP, Bourque C, Jones PJ, Ross R, Parsons WE, "Medium- versus long-chain triglycerides for 27 days increases fat oxidation and energy expenditure without resulting in changes in body composition in overweight women."
International Journal of Obesity and Related Metabolic Disorders. 2003 Jan; 27(1):95-102. DOI: 10.1038/sj.ijo.0802169.
https://www.ncbi.nlm.nih.gov/pubmed/12532160

17. St-Onge MP, Bosarge A, "Weight-loss diet that includes consumption of medium-chain triacylglycerol oil leads to a greater rate of weight and fat mass loss than does olive oil."

American Journal of Clinical Nutrition. 2008 Mar; 87(3):621-6.
DOI: 10.1093/ajcn/87.3.621.
www.ncbi.nlm.nih.gov/pubmed/18326600

18. Stubbs RJ, Harbron CG, "Covert manipulation of the ratio of medium- to long-chain triglycerides in isoenergetically dense diets: effect on food intake in ad libitum feeding men."
International Journal of Obesity and Related Metabolic Disorders. 1996 May; 20(5):435-44. PMID: 8696422.
www.ncbi.nlm.nih.gov/pubmed/8696422

19. Liau KM, Lee YY, Chen CK, Rasool AH, "An Open-Label Pilot Study to Assess the Efficacy and Safety of Virgin Coconut Oil in Reducing Visceral Adiposity."
ISRN Pharmacology. 2011 Mar 15; 2011: 949686. DOI: 10.5402/2011/949686.
www.ncbi.nlm.nih.gov/pubmed/22164340

20. Assunção ML, Ferreira HS, dos Santos AF, Cabral Jr CR, Florêncio TM, "Effects of dietary coconut oil on the biochemical and anthropometric profiles of women presenting abdominal obesity."
Lipids. 2009 Jul; 44(7):593-601. Epub 2009 May 13.
DOI: 10.1007/s11745-009-3306-6.
www.ncbi.nlm.nih.gov/pubmed/19437058

21. Laffel L, "Ketone bodies: a review of physiology, pathophysiology and application of monitoring to diabetes."
Diabetes/Metabolism Research and Reviews. 1999 Nov-Dec;15(6):412-26.
PMID: 10634967.
www.ncbi.nlm.nih.gov/pubmed/10634967

22. McCarty MF, DiNicolantonio JJ, "Lauric acid-rich medium-chain triglycerides can substitute for other oils in cooking applications and may have limited pathogenicity."
Open Heart. 2016 Jul 27; 3(2): e000467. DOI: 10.1136/openhrt-2016-000467.
www.ncbi.nlm.nih.gov/pmc/articles/PMC4975867

23. Enig MG, "Saturated Fats and the Lungs."
Online Article at: westonprice.org 2000 Jun 30.
www.westonaprice.org/health-topics/know-your-fats/saturated-fats-and-the-lungs/

DAY 16

1. www.oliveoilsource.com/page/chemical-characteristics

2. Menendez JA, Lupu R, "Mediterranean dietary traditions for the molecular treatment of human cancer: anti-oncogenic actions of the main olive oil's monounsaturated fatty acid oleic acid (18:1n-9)."
Current Pharmaceutical Biotechnology. 2006 Dec; 7(6):495-502. PMID: 17168666.
www.ncbi.nlm.nih.gov/pubmed/17168666

3. Menendez JA, Vellon L, Colomer R, Lupu R, "Oleic acid, the main monounsaturated fatty acid of olive oil, suppresses Her-2/neu (erbB-2) expression and synergistically enhances the growth inhibitory effects of trastuzumab (Herceptin) in breast cancer cells with Her-2/neu oncogene amplification."
Annals of Oncology. 2005 Mar; 16(3):359-71. DOI: 10.1093/annonc/mdi090.
www.ncbi.nlm.nih.gov/pubmed/15642702

4. Bes-Rastrollo M, Sánchez-Villegas A, de la Fuente C, de Irala J, Martinez JA, Martínez-González MA, "Olive oil consumption and weight change: the SUN prospective cohort study."
Lipids. 2006 Mar; 41(3):249-56. PMID: 16711599.
www.ncbi.nlm.nih.gov/pubmed/16711599

5. Razquin C, Martinez JA, Martinez-Gonzalez MA, Mitjavila MT, Estruch R, Marti A, "A 3 years follow-up of a Mediterranean diet rich in virgin olive oil is associated with high plasma antioxidant capacity and reduced body weight gain."
European Journal of Clinical Nutrition. 2009 Aug; (63)1387-1393.
DOI: 10.1038/ejcn.2009.106
www.nature.com/articles/ejcn2009106

6. Tin Win D, "Oleic Acid – the Anti-Breast Cancer Component in Olive Oil."
Assumption University Journal of Technology. 9(2): 75-78 (Oct. 2005).
Online PDF at:
www.aulibrary.au.edu/multim1/ABAC_Pub/Au-Journal-of-Technology/v9-n2-2.pdf

7. Garg A, "Adipose tissue dysfunction in obesity and lipodystrophy."
Clinical Cornerstone. 2006; 8 Suppl 4: S7-S13. PMID: 17208666.
www.ncbi.nlm.nih.gov/pubmed/17208666

8. Finucane OM, et al., "Monounsaturated fatty-acid-enriched high-fat diets impede adipose NLRP3 inflammasome-mediated IL-1B secretion and insulin resistance despite obesity."
Diabetes. 2015 June; 64(6):16-28. DOI: 10.2337/db14-1098.
www.ncbi.nlm.nih.gov/pubmed/25626736

9. Aller R, De Luis DA, Izaola O, de la Fuente B, Bachiller R, "Effect of a high monounsaturated vs high polyunsaturated fat hypocaloric diets in nonalcoholic fatty liver disease."
European Review for Medical and Pharmacological Sciences. 2014; 18(7):1041-7.
PMID: 24763885.
www.ncbi.nlm.nih.gov/pubmed/24763885

10. Yang JH, Chang JS, Chen CL, Yeh CL, Chien YW, "Effects of different amounts and types of dietary fatty acids on the body weight, fat accumulation, and lipid metabolism in hamsters."
Nutrition. 2016 May; 32(5): 601-8. DOI: 10.1016/j.nut.2015.11.010.
www.ncbi.nlm.nih.gov/pubmed/26896233

11. Fallon S, Enig MG, "The Great Con-ola."
Online Article at: westonprice.org 2002 Jul 28.
https://www.westonaprice.org/health-topics/know-your-fats/the-great-con-ola

12. Trenholm HL et al., "An Evaluation of the Relationship of Dietary Fatty Acids to Incidence of Myocardial Lesions in Male Rats."
Canadian Institute of Food Science Technology Journal. 1979 Oct; 12(4):189-193.
DOI: 10.1016/S0315-5463(79)73134-8.
www.sciencedirect.com/science/article/pii/S0315546379731348?via%3Dihub

13. Sauer FD et al., "Additional vitamin E required in milk replacer diets that contain canola oil."
Nutrition Research. 1997 Feb; 17(2):259-269.
DOI: 10.1016/S0271-5317(96)00256-4.
https://www.sciencedirect.com/science/article/pii/S0271531796002564

14. Kramer JK et al., "Hematological and lipid changes in newborn piglets fed milk-replacer diets containing erucic acid."
Lipids. 1998 Jan; 33(1):1-10. DOI: 10.1007/s11745-998-0174-1.
https://link.springer.com/article/10.1007/s11745-998-0174-1

DAY 17

1. Simopoulos AP, "The importance of the ratio of omega-6/omega-3 fatty acids."
Biomedicine & Pharmacotherapy. 2002 Oct; Volume 56, Issue 8, Pages 365-379.
DOI:10.1016/S0753-3322(02)00253-6.
www.sciencedirect.com/science/article/pii/S0753332202002536#!

2. Enig MG, Fallon SW, "The Oiling of America."
Online Article at: westonprice.org 2002 Jul 28.
https://www.westonaprice.org/health-topics/know-your-fats/the-great-con-ola/?option=com_content&view=article&id=525:the-oiling-of-america&-catid=32:know-your-fats&Itemid=134

3. Poonamjot D, Evans JR, Dhahbi J, Chellappa K, Han DS, Spindler S, Sladek FM, "Soybean Oil Is More Obesogenic and Diabetogenic than Coconut Oil and Fructose in Mouse; Potential Role for the Liver."
PLoS/One. 2015 July 22. DOI: 10.1371/journal.pone.0132672.
www.journals.plos.org/plosone/article?id=10.1371/journal.pone.0132672

4. Yang F, Zhang Y, Xu Q, Li R, Yang X, Liu Y, Wang J, Yu X, Xue C, "Effects of oils on lipid metabolism in obese C57BL/6J mice induced by a high fat diet."
Wei Sheng Yan Jiu. 2013 Nov; 42(6):901-6, 914. PMID: 24459899.
www.ncbi.nlm.nih.gov/pubmed/24459899

5. Patterson E, Wall R, Fitzgerald GF, Ross RP, Stanton C, "Health Implications of High Dietary Omega-6 Polyunsaturated Fatty Acids."
Journal of Nutrition and Metabolism. 2012 Apr 5; 2012:539426.DOI:

10.1155/2012/539426.
www.ncbi.nlm.nih.gov/pmc/articles/PMC3335257

6. Surette M, "The science behind dietary omega-3 fatty acids."
Canadian Medical Association Journal. 2008 Jan 15; 178(20: 177-180.
DOI: 10.1503/cmaj.071356.
www.ncbi.nlm.nih.gov/pmc/articles/PMC2174995

7. Kiecolt-Glaser JK, Belury MA, Porter K, Beversdorf DQ, Lemeshow S, Glaser R, "Depressive Symptoms, omega-6:omega-3 Fatty Acids, and Inflammation in Older Adults."
Psychosomatic Medicine. 2007 Apr; 69(3):217- 24.
DOI: 10.1097/PSY.0b013e3180313a45.
www.ncbi.nlm.nih.gov/pubmed/17401057

8. O'Keefe S, Gaskins-Wright S, Wiley V, Chen I-C, "Levels of *trans* geometrical isomer of essential fatty acids in some unhydrogenated U.S. vegetable oils."
Journal of Food Lipids. 1994 Sept; 1(3):165-176.
DOI: 10.1111/j.1745-4522.1994.tb00244.x.
www.onlinelibrary.wiley.com/doi/10.1111/j.1745-4522.1994.tb00244.x/abstract

9. Charles D, "The Forgotten, Fascinating Saga Of Crisco."
Online Article at: National Public Radio, Inc. 2012 Jan 9.
www.npr.org/sections/thesalt/2012/01/09/144918710/the-forgotten-fascinating-saga-of-crisco

10. Sircar S, Kansra U, "Choice of cooking oils --- myths and realities."
Journal of the Indian Medical Association. 1998 Oct; 96(10):304-7.
PMID: 10063298.
www.ncbi.nlm.nih.gov/pubmed/10063298

11. Mercola J, "Pine Nut Benefits: 5 Ways This Nutritious Seed Can Rejuvenate Your Body."
Online Article at: mercola.com 2015 Jan 19.
www.articles.mercola.com/sites/articles/archive/2015/01/19/pine-nuts-benefits.aspx

DAY 18

1. Conquer JA, Holub BJ, "Supplementation with an algae source of docosahexaenoic acid increases (n-3) fatty acid status and alters selected risk factors for heart disease in vegetarian subjects."
Journal of Nutrition. 1996 Dec; 126(12):3032-9. DOI: 10.1093/jn/126.12.3032.
www.ncbi.nlm.nih.gov/pubmed/9001371

2. Coad TL, "Difference Between Omega 3 & Algae Source."
Online Article at: livestrong.com (Accessed Nov 2018).
www.livestrong.com/article/494410-difference-between-omega-3-algae-source

3. Neubert AP, "Study: 3 square meals a day paired with lean protein help people feel full during weight loss."
Online Article at: Purdue University News Service 2011 Mar 30.
www.purdue.edu/newsroom/research/2011/110330CampbellPork.html

4. Cameron JD, Cyr MJ, Doucet E, "Increased meal frequency does not promote greater weight loss in subjects who were prescribed an 8-week equi-energetic energy-restricted diet."
British Journal of Nutrition. 2010 Apr; 103(8): 1098-101.
DOI: 10.1017/S0007114509992984.
www.ncbi.nlm.nih.gov/pubmed/19943985

5. DiGiulio S, "Experts Say This Diet Could Help You Lose Weight And Get More Sleep."
Online Article at: huffpost.com: Life/Healthy Living (Updated 2016 Apr 4).
www.huffingtonpost.com/entry/best-weight-loss-diet-for-sleep_us_56fd38a5e4b0a06d5804f282

6. Veldhorst MA, Westerterp-Plantenga MS, Westerterp KR, "Gluconeogenesis and energy expenditure after a high-protein, carbohydrate-free diet."
American Journal of Clinical Nutrition. 2009 Sep; 90(3):519-26.
DOI: 10.3945/ajcn.2009.27834.
www.ncbi.nlm.nih.gov/pubmed/19640952

7. Johnston CS, Day CS, Swan PD, "Postprandial thermogenesis is increased 100% on a high-protein, low-fat diet versus a high-carbohydrate, low-fat diet in healthy, young women."
Journal of the American College of Nutrition. 2002 Feb; 21(1):55-61.
PMID: 11838888.
www.ncbi.nlm.nih.gov/pubmed/11838888

8. Veldhorst MA, Westerterp KR, van Vught AJ, Westerter_Plantenga MS, "Presence or absence of carbohydrates and the proportion of fat in a high-protein diet affect appetite suppression but not energy expenditure in normal-weight human subjects fed in energy balance."
British Journal of Nutrition. 2010 Nov; 104(9):1395-405.
DOI: 10.1017/S0007114510002060.
www.ncbi.nlm.nih.gov/pubmed/20565999

9. Johnstone AM, Stubbs RJ, Harbron CG, "Effect of overfeeding macronutrients on day-to-day food intake in man."
European Journal of Clinical Nutrition. 1996 Jul; 50(7):418-30. PMID: 8862477.
www.ncbi.nlm.nih.gov/pubmed/8862477

10. Halton TL, Hu FB, "The effects of high protein diets on thermogenesis, satiety and weight loss: a critical review."
Journal of the American College of Nutrition. 2004 Oct; 23(5):373-85.
PMID: 15466943.
www.ncbi.nlm.nih.gov/pubmed/15466943

DAY 19

11. Mercola J, "Your Practical Guide to Omega-3 Benefits and Supplementation."
Online Article at: mercola.com (Accessed July 2018).
https://articles.mercola.com/omega-3.aspx

DAY 19

1. Gao Z, Yin J, Zhang J, Ward RE, Marin RJ, Lefevre M, Cefalu WT, Ye J, "Butyrate improves insulin sensitivity and increases energy expenditure in mice."
Diabetes. 2009 Jul; 58(7):1509017. DOI: 10.2337/db08-1637.
www.ncbi.nlm.nih.gov/pubmed/19366864

2. Masterjohn C, "Saturated Fat Does a Body Good."
Online Article at: The Weston A. Price Foundation 2016 May 6.
www.westonaprice.org/health-topics/abcs-of-nutrition/saturated-fat-body-good

3. Rolland V, Roseau S, Gromentin G, Nicolaidis S, Tomé D, Even PC, "Body weight, body composition, and energy metabolism in lean and obese Zucker rats fed soybean oil or butter."
American Journal of Clinical Nutrition. 2002 Jan 1; 75:21–30.
DOI: 10.1093/ajcn/75.1.21.
https://academic.oup.com/ajcn/article/75/1/21/4689241

4. Siri-Tarino PW, Chiu S, Bergeron N, Krauss RM, "Saturated Fats Versus Polyunsaturated Fats Versus Carbohydrates for Cardiovascular Disease Prevention and Treatment."
Annual Review of Nutrition. 2015; 35: 517–543.
DOI: 10.1146/annurev-nutr-071714-034449.
www.ncbi.nlm.nih.gov/pmc/articles/PMC4744652
There is growing evidence that SFAs in the context of dairy foods, particularly fermented dairy products, have neutral or inverse associations with CVD [Cardio Vascular Disease].

5. Blesso CN, Andersen CJ, Barona J, Volek JS, Fernandez ML, "Whole egg consumption improves lipoprotein profiles and insulin sensitivity to a greater extent than yolk-free egg substitute in individuals with metabolic syndrome."
Metabolism. 2013 Mar; 62(3):400-10. DOI: 10.1016/j.metabol.2012.08.014.
www.ncbi.nlm.nih.gov/pubmed/23021013

DAY 20

1. Kris-Etherton PM, Griel AE, Psota TL, et al. "Dietary stearic acid and risk of cardiovascular disease: Intake, sources, digestion, and absorption."
Lipids. 2005 Dec; 40: 1193. DOI: 10.1007/s11745-005-1485-y.
link.springer.com/article/10.1007/s11745-005-1485-y

2. "Stearic Acid"
Online Article at: beefresearch.org (Accessed Dec 2018).

(Research Knowledge & Management/Human Nutrition Research PDF)
https://www.beefresearch.org/CMDocs/BeefResearch/Nutrition_Fact_Sheets/Stearic_Acid.pdf

3. Grundy SM, "Influence of stearic acid on cholesterol metabolism relative to other long-chain fatty acids."
American Journal of Clinical Nutrition. 1994 Dec; 60(6 Suppl): 986S-990S.
DOI: 10.1093/ajcn/60.6.986S.
www.ncbi.nlm.nih.gov/pubmed/7977157

4. Mensink RP, "Effects of stearic acid on plasma lipid and lipoproteins in humans."
Lipids. 2005 Dec; 40(12):1201-5. PMID: 16477803.
www.ncbi.nlm.nih.gov/pubmed/16477803

5. "Proteins: What's the Recommended Intake?"
Online Article at: mercola.com
www.mercola.com/nutritionplan/beginner_proteins.htm

6. Bendsen N T, Christensen R, Martels EM, Astrup A, "Consumption of industrial and ruminant trans fatty acids and risk of coronary heart disease: a systematic review and meta-analysis of cohort studies."
European Journal of Clinical Nutrition. 2011 Mar 23; 65, 773-783 (2011).
DOI: 10.1038/ejcn.2011.34.
www.europepmc.org/abstract/med/21427742

7. Rainer L, Heiss CJ, "Conjugated linoleic acid: health implications and effects on body composition."
Journal of the American Dietetic Association. 2004 Jun; Vol 104, Issue 8, Pages 963-968.
www.sciencedirect.com/science/article/pii/S0002822304004316#

8. Gaullier JM, Halse J, Høye K, Kristiansen K, Fagertun H, Vik H, Gudmundsen O, "Supplementation with Conjugated Linoleic Acid for 24 Months Is Well Tolerated by and Reduces Body Fat Mass in Healthy, Overweight Humans."
The Journal of Nutrition. 2005 Apr; Volume 135, Issue 4, Pages 778–784.
DOI: 10.1093/jn/135.4.778.
www.academic.oup.com/jn/article/135/4/778/4663753

9. Rahman Md M, Halade GV, Jamali A El, Fernandes G, "Conjugated linoleic acid (CLA) prevents age associated skeletal muscle loss."
Biochemical and Biophysical Research Communications. 2009 Jun 12; 383(40):513-518. DOI: 10.1016/j.bbrc.2009.04.071.
www.ncbi.nlm.nih.gov/pmc/articles/PMC2893570

10. Nicklas TA, O'Neil CE, Zanovec M, Keast D, Fulgoni VL III. "Contribution of beef consumption to nutrient intake, diet quality, and food patterns in the diets of the US population."
Meat Science. 2012 Jan; 90:152-8. DOI: 10.1016/j.meatsci.2011.06.021.
www.ncbi.nlm.nih.gov/pubmed/21752554

11. O'Neil CE, Keast DR, Nicklas TA, Fulgoni VL, "Food sources of energy and nutrients among adults in the US: NHANES 2003-2006."
Nutrients. 2012 Dec 19; 4(12):2097-2120. DOI: 10.3390/nu4122097.
www.ncbi.nlm.nih.gov/pubmed/23363999

DAY 21

1. Jakobsen MU, Dethlefsen C, Joensen AM, Stegger J, Tjonneland A, et al., "Intake of carbohydrates compared with intake of saturated fatty acids and risk of myocardial infarction: importance of the glycemic index."
American Journal of Clinical Nutrition. 2010 Jun; 91:1764–68.
DOI: 10.3945/ajcn.2009.29099.
www.ncbi.nlm.nih.gov/pubmed/20375186

2. Micha R, Mozaffarian D, "Saturated fat and cardiometabolic risk factors, coronary heart disease, stroke, and diabetes: a fresh look at the evidence."
Lipids. 2010 Oct; 45:893–905. DOI: 10.1007/s11745-010-3393-4.
www.ncbi.nlm.nih.gov/pmc/articles/PMC2950931

3. Samsel A, Seneff S, "Glyphosate's Suppression of Cytochrome P450 Enzymes and Amino Acid Biosynthesis by the Gut Microbiome: Pathways to Modern Diseases."
Entropy. 2013; 15(4), 1416-1463; doi:10.3390/e15041416.
DOI: 10.3390/e15041416.
www.mdpi.com/1099-4300/15/4/1416

4. Hyman M, *The Blood Sugar Solution* (2012). Little Brown and Company: New York NY

5. Davis W, *Wheat Belly: Lose the Wheat, Lose the Weight, and Find Your Path Back to Health* (2014). Rodale Publishing: Emmaus, PA

6. Eslick, GD; "Gastrointestinal symptoms and obesity: A meta-analysis."
Obesity Reviews. 2012 May; 13(5):469-79. DOI: 10.1111/j.1467-789X.2011.00969.x.
www.ncbi.nlm.nih.gov/pubmed/22188520

7. Yu JC, Berger P3rd., "Sleep apnea and obesity."
South Dakota Medicine. 2011; Spec No: 28-34. PMID: 21717814.
www.ncbi.nlm.nih.gov/pubmed/21717814

BONUS DAY

1. Barnosky AR, Hoddy KK, Unterman TG, Varady KA, "Intermittent fasting vs daily calorie restriction for type 2 diabetes prevention: a review of human findings."
(In-Depth Review Article: *Excess Adiposity and Disease*).
2014 Oct; Volume 164, Issue 4, Pages 302-311.
DOI: 10.1016/j.trsl.2014.05.013.
www.sciencedirect.com/science/article/pii/S193152441400200X

2. Antoni R, Johnston KL, Collins AL, Robertson MD, "The Effects of Intermittent Energy Restriction on Indices of Cardiometabolic Health."
Research in Endocrinology. 2014 Jun 28; Vol. 2014, Article ID 459119.
DOI: 10.5171/2014.459119.
www.ibimapublishing.com/articles/ENDO/2014/459119/

3. Longo VD, Mattson MP, "Fasting: Molecular Mechanisms and Clinical Applications."
Cell Metabolism. 2014 Feb 4; 19(20: 181-192. DOI: 10.1016/j.cmet.2013.12.008.
www.ncbi.nlm.nih.gov/pmc/articles/PMC3946160

4. Heilbronn LK, Smith SR, Martin CK, Anton SD, Ravussin E, "Alternate-day fasting in nonobese subjects: effects on body weight, body composition, and energy metabolism."
American Journal of Clinical Nutrition. 2005 Jan; 81(1):69-73.
DOI: 10.1093/ajcn/81.1.69.
www.ncbi.nlm.nih.gov/pubmed/15640462

5. Zauner C, Schneeweiss B, Kranz A, Madl C, Ratheiser K, Kramer L, Roth E, Schneider B, Lenz K, "Resting energy expenditure in short-term starvation is increased as a result of an increase in serum norepinephrine."
American Journal of Clinical Nutrition. 2000 Jun; 71(16):1511-5.
DOI: 10.1093/ajcn/71.6.1511.
www.ncbi.nlm.nih.gov/pubmed/10837292

6. Varady KA, "Intermittent versus daily calorie restriction: which diet regimen is more effective for weight loss?"
Obesity Reviews. 2011 Jul; 12(7): e593-601. DOI: 10.1111/j.1467-789X.2011.00873.x.
www.ncbi.nlm.nih.gov/pubmed/21410865

7. Grassi D, Lippi C, Necozione S, Desideri G, Ferri C, "Short-term administration of dark chocolate is followed by a significant increase in insulin sensitivity and a decrease in blood pressure in healthy persons."
American Journal of Clinical Nutrition. 2005 Mar; 81(3):611-4.
DOI: 10.1093/ajcn/81.3.611.
www.ncbi.nlm.nih.gov/pubmed/15755830

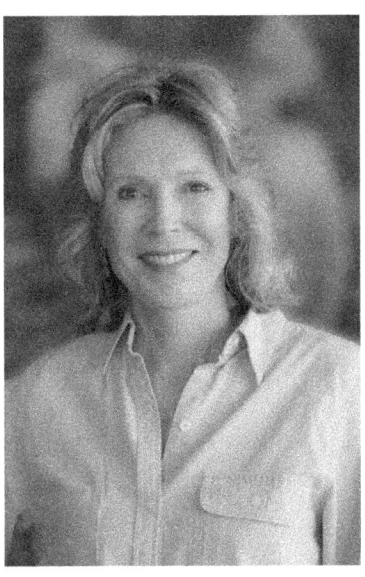

Kris Doran Williams is a Master Certified Health Coach with the Dr. Sears Wellness Institute.
She is committed to helping others seek the Truth --- for this life and the next.
She is also committed to helping anyone who wants to live a healthy and productive life gain a better understanding of Dr. Sears' four principles of health: Lifestyle, Exercise, Attitude, and Nutrition. For more information and personalized coaching, please go to
www.kriswilliamswellness.com.

Has this guide helped you in any way that you think will benefit others? Please let them know by writing your review of this book online at your site of purchase.

www.ingramcontent.com/pod-product-compliance
Lightning Source LLC
Chambersburg PA
CBHW020245030426
42336CB00010B/620